View from the
Bedpan

VIEW
from the
BEDPAN

**A candid look at
hospitalization and healing**

BEVERLEY JUNE RICHMOND

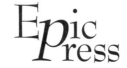

Epic
Press

Belleville, Ontario, Canada

View from the Bedpan

Copyright © 2002, Beverley Richmond

Second Printing: April 2003

**For more information or
to order additional copies, please contact:**

Beverley Richmond
RR#1 Hillier, ON
Canada, KOK 2JO
(613) 399-3696

National Library of Canada Cataloguing in Publication

Richmond, Beverley, 1951-
    View from the bedpan : a candid look at hospitalization and healing / Beverley Richmond.

ISBN 1-55306-361-9

    1. Hospital patients. 2. Hospital care. I. Title.

RA965.6.R52 2002   362.1'1   C2002-902228-2

Epic Press is an imprint of *Essence Publishing*. For more information, contact:
20 Hanna Court, Belleville, Ontario, Canada K8P 5J2.
Phone: 1-800-238-6376. Fax: (613) 962-3055.
E-mail: publishing@essencegroup.com
Internet: www.essencegroup.com

Printed in Canada
by

To the many nurses, doctors, surgeons,
hospital personnel, and health care workers,
who each and every day dedicate themselves
to saving and rebuilding lives.

To devoted family members and friends,
who, as attentive caregivers,
make possible the most remarkable healing.

To survivors who have learned the hard way that
extraordinary people are made, not born,
and miracles happen every day.

～ Table of Contents ～

Acknowledgments. 9

Preface 11

Introduction 17

Part I—The Bedpan

The Accident. 25

Intensive Care. 30

Critical Care 33

Hallucinations 35

Hospital "Ladies". 38

Visitors 41

Hemorrhoids and Other Matters 45

The Dining Room. 48

Menopause or MVA? (Motor Vehicle Accident) 50

Interesting People 52

The Weekend Pass 55

Others' Reactions. 58

Cards and Letters. 60

Depression, Loneliness, Isolation 64

Excuse Me, May I Please Have the Rest
of My Skull Back? 68

Part II—The View

The Nurses 87

Jargon 92

Spouse and Caregiver 95

The Closed Door 99

"If Only I Hadn't" Syndrome 101

Shared Experiences 103

Roommates. 107

Fears and Phobias 110

The Brick Wall—Exhaustion 115

The Injuries. 116

The Pain—Blockout 124

Therapists 126

Hair 131

Philosophy and Religion 140

The Dream—Accident Revisited. 142

Part III—Final Notes

In Retrospect. 151

Appendix—Strategies and Suggestions

Hospital Strategies. 159

Patient Checklist. 162

Visitor and Caregiver Checklist 164

✑ Acknowledgments ✑

View from the Bedpan had many helpers along the way, either through their direct input or ongoing expressed confidence in me. "Thank you" goes to:

My parents Lillian and William Richmond, for telling me as a child that I had "a way with words."

My friend and partner Doug Hebbel, for reminding me to "write it down," and for acting as my memory when my own memory failed.

Clinical psychologist Dr. Carol Harris, for helping me define who I could be in my new post-accident life, and for offering ongoing support and interest in the development of this book.

Author Janet Lunn, Order of Canada, and poet Louise O'Donnell for their kind words of encouragement to "keep writing."

John Kumpf, the executive director of the Ontario Brain Injury Association, whose enthusiasm spurred me on through many hesitant moments.

Freelance editors Jane Karchmar and Marjorie Green, and General Store Publishing House publisher Tim Gordon, for their comments that helped shape the manuscript and instilled confidence in me for this project.

Carole Vincent, founder of the Brain Injury Association Quinte District and also a survivor caregiver, whose own experiences and those of her son, Randy, helped validate my written words.

Mrs. Darlington, for her constructive literary and artistic comments.

All those at Essence Publishing, who designed, polished, and brought my book to its completion.

And, a large cast of nurses, doctors, and health care professionals for their essential role in my survival, without which, of course, this book would be impossible.

∾ Preface ∾

YOU COULD CALL ME A PROFESSIONAL PATIENT. I'VE BEEN IN and out of hospitals all my life. The most recent visits were in 1992 for open-heart valve replacement surgery, and in 1994/95 following a near-fatal motor vehicle accident that resulted in orthopedic and brain injuries. This book was written from personal experiences, observations, and impressions made in the hospital after the accident and after my return home to recuperate.

Having always been an inquisitive person with a different perspective, a sense of humour, and an optimistic outlook, those traits didn't leave me when I entered the hospital. There I observed how vulnerable, lonely, and miserable most of the hospital patients around me appeared to be. Like me, they were sick or injured, but, on a positive note, the majority of us were there *to get well*. And everyone seemed so scared, not knowing what to expect, and not questioning or confiding in others around them.

I felt they needed a private way to share their thoughts, experiences, anxieties, and joys. So I thought about writing a book which could provide that outlet, and at the same time provide encouragement, help, and amusement to its readers.

After I was released from the hospital, post-accident, I visited several stores in search of a book to compare my hospital experiences with those of others. My search revealed only one small-print book on the hospital experience, a book I found to be cold, technical, alarming, and unreadable.

When it became obvious I wouldn't be returning to work because of my permanent injuries, I wrote this book. As well as relating my own personal thoughts, emotions, and experiences—the ups and downs of body, mind, and spirit—this book hopes to act as a "hospital helper," giving tips on how I survived the ordeal and how others can too. Often philosophical, it offers insights into various aspects of illness; at other times it records poignant moments. It suggests ways to cope with the hospital experience by finding the humour in it and by offering hope and inspiration. It's a known fact that humour speeds the recovery process.

For caregivers who want to help but aren't sure how, this book provides tips on what and what not to do in making the patient's hospital stay more bearable. Medical staff and students will find it a revealing look at hospitalization and healing from the patient's viewpoint; often, it's a tribute to nurses.

The book is a collection of stand-alone chapters written at various stages of my recovery. The first chapter I wrote—the one on depression and loneliness—was written five months following the accident; some chapters were written three years after.

At first I didn't keep a health journal, but later at the advice of my lawyer, I kept one religiously. In some places I drew or quoted from the journal, whereas other chapters I wrote from memory; some chapters were written as the events were happening.

During my recovery, I went through various phases of mental and physical well-being and not-so-well-being. These stages reveal themselves throughout the book. The ongoing struggle I endured while writing was the lack of stamina—physical, mental, and emotional—during the entire period. In times of tremendous change and personal difficulty, spiritual beliefs are either challenged or developed; you will read that mine were no exception.

I tried to end most chapters on an up beat, with helpful tips or perhaps a summarizing thought. However, not all chapters or subjects lent themselves to this format; not all chapters had happy endings. The reason, of course, is that hospital life is like Life, and, accordingly, has both good and bad experiences. The need to share our hospital experiences seems to be universal; this book offers you a safe way to do that.

The book is topic-oriented; I believe this format allows you the option of using it as a handbook. When read from start to finish the book relates an interesting journey. I've tried to include everything: the coping, the agony, the laughs, the complications, the sharing, the frustration, the caring, the compassion, and the many small victories.

It will become clear to the reader that we are not alone in our suffering or our healing. There are a multitude of people who play a major, vital role. Loved ones, hospital staff, health service providers, and all our acquaintances contribute in so many ways to our recovery process. I've tried to acknowledge and thank many of these groups for their efforts.

Hopefully, this book will help console, heal, inform, inspire, guide, and amuse you. Perhaps it will:

- inspire some patients to laugh at their predicament, thereby promoting healing by seeing their situation in a different light;

- relieve some feelings of anxiety and loneliness;

- provide a private way to share hospital experiences;

- offer ideas on what to expect as a daily routine as a hospital patient;

- suggest ways to make the most of the patient's hospital stay;

- encourage interaction between patients;

- provide an interesting account of one woman's accident and her journey back to wellness through struggle and change;

- help family caregivers and friends do the right thing for their hospitalized loved ones;

- inform the medical profession about how it feels to be hospital-bound, and about life after release;

- educate the healthcare industry about what it's doing right and wrong;

- contribute further information on brain injury and its consequences;

- pay tribute to hospitals, nurses, and to those patients who demonstrate daily the human spirit and capacity for survival.

In closing, my goal is that all readers—whether hospital

patients (past, present, or future), doctors, nurses, medical students, psychologists, hospital administrators and staff, the friends and family of patients, those curious about the hospital experience, or those curious about the experiences of one particular woman—will find this a useful, engaging book.

Illness and hospitalization are like any other part of life: multi-dimensional and multi-experiential. Ideally, this little book reflects that. I hope you enjoy it.

∾ INTRODUCTION ∾

I THINK EARLY CHILDHOOD PREPARED ME FOR WHAT WOULD happen approximately forty years later.

Going back in time I vaguely remember a large room filled with many people. There, I would wait with my mother and sister until a friendly lady (nurse) came for us. I wasn't sick. My sister, who was five years older than I, had tuberculosis in her finger bone. The doctor told Mom they could save my sister's finger from amputation if she was prepared to bring her to the hospital for a needle every week for a year. Being the little one, I tagged along, and while my sister got shots to eliminate the disease, I got serum shots to test if I had developed it. Mom saved my sister's finger, and I had obtained my first remembered hospital experiences.

When older I remember going to the hospital for surgery on my left eye; a ptosis operation they called it. I had droopy eyelids that interfered somewhat with my vision. My parents sometimes teased me that I was a Chinese baby; I wondered about the milkman a lot.

Later on I had the other eye done, and years later I would be back in the hospital to have the second one done again.

When I was about fifteen, I entered a Toronto hospital for a special test that involved injecting dye into my bloodstream, so doctors could observe its circulation throughout my heart and body. In preparation, I remember taking a tepid bath in a large cold room with a huge floor-to-ceiling picture window, sans curtain, overlooking busy University Avenue. I wondered if anyone was looking up at me from below or from offices on the other side of the wide boulevard.

Later in the operating room, a burning flush swept through me as the dye made its rounds, jolting me aware of every blood vessel in my body. I remember being strapped to a table that tilted to the left, then to the right. I was afraid I'd fall off, but the safety straps held. This testing was being done because doctors suspected a heart murmur.

On Christmas Eve the phone call came. The doctor said I had a hole in my heart (as they called it in those days) and I could die. He went on to say that the mitral valve leak was a birth defect, and I might need surgery in the future. That sounded a lot better than dying.

In my early twenties, I decided my Canadian nose, reminiscent of its Polish/Ukrainian/English heritage, was a little too bumpy and a little too bulbous to be seen on my petite face and frame, so I underwent surgery to reduce the bulbous tip and remove the Roman bump. Although not as chiseled and refined as I would have liked, the result was an improvement.

Without my realizing it, what had been happening to me was a series of positive reinforcement hospital experiences designed to bolster my confidence in hospitals, and help prepare me for what was to come.

Another hospital visit in my early twenties left an impact. At the tender age of twenty-eight, my sister Barb suffered a brain aneurysm. I remember visiting her shortly after her nine-hour life-saving surgery, gazing down at the white bandage encircling the top half of her skull and looking into her eyes—those vacant, unremembering eyes staring up at me in their emptiness. To this day that image haunts me. Mother again nurtured Barb back to health; her daily visits, first to the general hospital and then to the rehab hospital, helped Barb return home to her husband.

I had just turned forty, and had endured ten years of struggle holding down a hectic career at Harbourfront while helping run my husband's struggling retail business, which eventually failed. It was time to make a drastic lifestyle change. Putting all that stress and disappointment behind, we moved far away to begin a peaceful, positive, simple life in a small rural community. My newly found employment in advertising sales at the city newspaper, a wonderful job I loved, proved to be another level of stress.

Two years later my heart began to fail; I got weaker daily. After much testing, doctors decided it was time for surgery. I now had two leaky valves to replace—the mitral and also the aortic. Surgery was scheduled, then postponed, then rescheduled and postponed. Nine months passed while I was knocked further and further down the waiting list, as emergency surgery took precedence over elective surgery. As far as I was concerned, my surgery was an emergency, not elective.

The stress of waiting proved too much; my health was going downhill fast. One day in desperation, feeling extremely weak and frightened, I phoned the surgery scheduling coordinator and, in a crying fit, secured a firm surgery date two weeks away. When the August '92 admitting day arrived, just before leaving for the hospital Doug took photos of me and the hounds just in case I didn't return.

The surgery went well, for the most part. After seven days they decided to send me home. I thought about refusing to go because something seemed horribly wrong. My abdomen was extremely distended, which wasn't normal for me, I kept telling the nurses. It didn't seem to matter what I said; the doctors sent me home anyway.

Over the next nine days my condition worsened. On the tenth day, feeling extremely ill, I told the visiting Home Care nurse I thought I should be back in hospital. After taking my vitals and consulting with my family doctor, the nurse agreed. I was taken to the city hospital for tests and monitoring, then rushed to the regional hospital by ambulance for emergency surgery. My body wasn't absorbing the post-surgery fluids from around the heart area, and they were collecting dangerously in the pericardium sac. Surgeons removed the fluids, and seven days later I was sent back home again to heal.

Understandably, it's at this point I developed an aversion to hospitals. My confidence in hospitals, doctors, and the medical system was uprooted. I learned there is only one person who has the patient's best interests as top priority—the patient himself. I also decided a proactive approach to "patient-hood" was absolutely necessary for survival. That had been proven to me. So, from then on, I became a pro-active patient.

Up until now, it may seem like I've spent a lifetime in and out of hospitals. As it turned out, I'd only spent half a lifetime.

Little did I know that two years later, in December '94, mechanical heart valves and all, I would nearly die under the wheels of a van. That accident, in more ways than one, started my second lifetime by ending most semblance of it to the past. I was also fast becoming a professional patient, and, as such, my *View from the Bedpan* begins.

The Bedpan

❧ The Accident

On Wednesday, December 21, 1994 at 10:25 a.m. I learned never to tempt fate.

It was a very busy time at the paper. Pre-Christmas advertising was almost wrapped up, and Boxing Day promotions were the main focus. As the downtown advertising rep, I was working my way up the main street calling on retailers, gathering orders and copy for their Boxing Day ads.

It was a cold, dry day, yet warm enough to sport a pair of black pumps with my raspberry-red, full-length wool coat. I loved that coat. Big, baggy, and straight-cut it was like walking around bundled in a warm, woolen blanket. It was functional, yet sophisticated—a little like myself, I mused.

I crossed to the other side and headed back down the street to call on the other half of the downtown retailers. Someone called out my name, and when I turned I saw a familiar face. It was Romano, a fellow advertising rep, who once worked at the newspaper but now worked for a competitor. He called me over.

We chatted about this and that, and then I asked about his wife. He told me she had injured her wrist over a year ago while skating, but she was still having problems heal-ing. We talked a bit more, and a little later as we said our good-byes and Merry Christmas, I added, "Isn't it funny how you go along and, suddenly, one day 'wham' some-thing happens that changes your life forever."

With that innocent comment, I had tempted fate. I turned and walked to the curb to continue my route down street. The light turned green, the little man in the traffic lights said walk, I looked both ways, then stepped off the curb. I remember thinking about Christmas gifts yet to buy. When I reached halfway across the intersection I looked up at the green walk signal one more time. I would remember little from then on.

The turning, full-size van hit my right side, knocking me 20 feet through the air, and then ran over me as I landed on the road. An off-duty OPP officer, who was making the same turn directly behind the van, saw the accident, stopped, and ran into the nearby police station to get help. An unidentified shopper exiting the jewellery store across the street, saw me fly through the air after being struck, and hurried back inside to phone the ambulance.

At the same time Al, the off-duty Town Crier, was walking up the street nearing the intersection when he heard a thud; there, ahead on the cold winter street, I lay dead still. Al stopped in his tracks and hurried into the nearest store, the bakery, to get help. He and Jane, the bakery owner, grabbed a blanket and ran to the accident scene. While they placed the blanket carefully over me, others got involved straightening my clothes, and yet another three onlookers removed their winter coats and placed them over me for added warmth.

Sandra from the beauty school across the street, who was also a part-time mailroom worker at the newspaper, ·joined the gathering crowd and knelt beside me on the ground, stroking my head and soothing me. "Where am I?" they say I asked, but I don't remember asking this. "What happened?" they say I asked, but I don't remember asking this either.

The little I do remember was this:

I was aware of lying on the hard ground, sensing a crowd of people around me. They were faceless from where I lay and everything was a blur. Someone was soothing me, stroking my head. Then I heard the words, "Beverley, this is Jane from the bakery. The ambulance has been called and Doug is on his way up from Picton."

"Is this a dream or is this really happening?" I drawled.

"No, Beverley, this isn't a dream. This is really happening."

"Where's my briefcase?"

"Your briefcase is here."

"Where's my ruler?"

"Your ruler's here too."

Slowly, I became aware of a wet, sticky, uncomfortable feeling in the middle of my right coat sleeve. When someone in the crowd yelled out, "Look at the tire tracks down her!" I began thinking something was horribly wrong. A wave of dread washed over me, followed by a sinking weakness. Something terrible had happened....

That was all I would remember for several days.

Meanwhile, the crowd set its sights on the driver of the van. Some formed a line in front of it, blocking any potential getaway; another held onto the van door in case the driver planned to run. "She (the driver) thought she had killed you," Martin, from the comic-book store, later told me.

As the police poured out of the nearby station, the witnesses and onlookers stood pointing their fingers in the driver's direction. Even the bank tellers from behind the huge windows were pointing, motioning at the van. There was no doubt in anybody's mind who had hit me.

Oblivious to all of this, I was still asking questions.

"Where's my ruler?"

"It's here, too," came the response, although this one stumped the onlookers. Ruler? They wondered out loud and looked at each other in confusion. Why was I asking about something so unimportant as a ruler? How could they know the ruler in question was a necessary tool of my trade? How could I sell ads if I couldn't measure and quote on them? They say I also asked, "Where's my calculator?" but I don't remember asking that.

Jane reflects that I was lying there very straight and calm on the roadway, as if gathering all my strength and resources together, shaking my head from side to side and repeating over and over, "I don't want to die. I don't want to die. I don't want to die...."

They say I also began to repeat, "Tell the doctors I'm on blood thinners." To this date I have no recollection of any of this, and am amazed at my composure and presence of mind under such extreme trauma. Incredible what the mind does when its survival is threatened.

"It was over in about five to ten minutes," reflects Martin.

"It all happened so quickly, so efficiently, as if everyone had a role to play," remembers Jane. "Everything went so smoothly."

The ambulance came, put me on the trauma board, taped my head and neck brace to it, while the newspaper photographer (not knowing the victim was me, a co-worker) clicked a photo, then was off. I was rushed to BGH emergency where my vitals were monitored. After assessing the injuries—too much for them to handle—I was rushed to KGH. I didn't hear the sirens, or remember the ambulance drivers, or the ride. Nothing.

Meanwhile, back downtown, something very strange happened. After the ambulance carrying me left the accident scene and the crowd dispersed, three ladies wandered into the bakery, each at different times, and strangely each one said independently to Jane, "She looked like a little angel lying there."

I must have been close to being an angel myself, that is, dying, but how close I was I'll never know. Surely, if there was an angel involved, it was my guardian angel.

At Kingston General my broken arm, broken leg, and broken head and brain were mended by a team of neuro and orthopedic surgeons. They didn't know if I'd live or not. Due to the blood thinners I was taking to prevent clots forming on my heart valves, there were major bleeding complications. After opening my skull to access my brain, they had to pack it and chemically immobilize me until they brought the bleeding under enough control for surgery.

News of my accident spread quickly throughout the downtown. The three "angel" ladies visited the bakery in the days ahead, to chat with Jane and catch up on my condition. I'm positive it was caring interest like this and the power of many prayers that helped me live through the crisis.

Analyzing later what happened to me, what's really interesting is that some bits of information are remembered, while others are forgotten, and still others were fabricated by me.

For example, I now know no one said to me, "Doug is on his way up from Picton," because no one in the crowd knew I had a Doug, nor that he worked in Picton. I can only surmise my mind created this coping technique out of a little wishful thinking.

One year later I was still putting together events, like pieces to a jigsaw puzzle. While the majority of details and experiences were remembered or gleaned from friends and witnesses shortly after the accident, I occasionally bump into someone who was there that day; their new details help shed more light on the events that will, for some time, and perhaps forever, remain somewhat of a mystery to me.

Many months following my release from hospital, upon returning for a routine ECG, the lab technician commented, "You're in a lot better condition than the last time I saw you." Desperately wanting more details, I asked if she was on duty the day I was brought into emergency. "What was it like? Can you tell me about it?"

"It was a long time ago," she tried to remember. "You were out of control, a little wild," she said with a smile.

Having no recollection of that either, she had given me yet another piece to my puzzle.

❧ Intensive Care

Christmas Eve, Saturday, December 24, 1994...

Behind the double doors of Intensive Care I lay, a tiny figure covered with a white sheet, arms sticking out from under it, hooked up to a ventilator, with wires, and hoses, and monitors beeping, and doctors and nurses coming and going.

The doctor squeezes my hand and says hello. No response. I'm aware, but not awake. He tells my friends to speak to me, for although I don't talk, I'm aware of things going on around me. (I may be aware, but I don't remember one thing.) Jeff and Heather speak to me; my eyes are closed and I give no response. Jeff kisses me on the cheek and I feel the brush of a soft beard. I sense it's him, but I'm not sure. Then they leave.

My first recollection must have been of this day. I'm still not sure what happened, but I try to put the pieces together in an effort to figure it all out.

Doing this was hard, with little to go on—only an awareness of unrecognizable faces being thrust close to mine, muffled voices, a kiss on the cheek or lips, a hand held or squeezed. That was all. There was no recollection of doctors, nurses, wires, hoses, tubes, ventilators, monitors, IVs, voices, beeping… nothing.

My mother always keeps a pen and paper beside the telephone to jot down notes during phone conversations; her talks with Doug were no exception. Without her notes I'd have no chronological record of those first few days.

Her staccato jottings described a cacophony of events. Here are Mom's records of Doug's daily calls updating her of my condition:

Wed., Dec. 21/94:
Beverley. Ran over by van this morning. Broken leg. Broken elbow. Blood behind ear. Loose teeth. 3:20 p.m. Doug's waiting for ferry over to Kingston Hospital. Blood thinner pills. Doug'll phone tonight. Please phone sister Barb/Ken.

Thurs., Dec. 22/94:
Set leg and elbow. Operated on skull. Blood thinner big problem. 4-7 days ICU expected.

Fri., Dec. 23/94:

Take bandage off head. Swelling on face down. CAT scan. Heart cardiogram. Respirator off. Neck brace. Positive.

Sun., Dec. 25/94:

Waken up at Christmas. Hands strength. Flexes toes up and down. Sitting up on a little angle. Left eye. Breathing tube in mouth.

Mon., Dec. 26/94:

Breathing tube out. Respirator off. Very restless. Stella caught a skunk. [This more humourous note was about my grey-hound and her encounter in the drive shed back home.]

Tues., Dec. 27/94:

Bandages off. Just small patch of hair shaved off part of head. Gets restless and kicks blankets off. Oxygen for breathing. Pumping blood medication. Hands restrained. Wears cervical collar. Asked for sister at 4:00 a.m.

In Intensive Care I had my own nurse whose job it was to sit at the end of the bed watching every move I made, night and day. I wasn't special: everyone in ICU had his or her own nurse; if we didn't, we'd probably not survive.

"The ICU nurses were fast!" recalls Doug. They often responded with impressive speed to grab my arm mid-air, as I tried to yank out the breathing tube. After Monday my hands needed to be restrained, because in my morphine stupor I had become extremely restless, determined to break free, to get away, to escape.

The next day they moved me out of Intensive Care into the Critical Care Unit. This meant I would share a nurse with other patients, and, for the most part, I was out of life-and-death danger.

∾ Critical Care

My mother's notes of Doug's daily phone calls to update her on my condition continue...

Wed., Dec. 28/94:
Out of ICU. Now in Neurology Critical Care head injury unit. Closely monitored. Cast. Catheter. Memory good. Do not cry, sister. Blood thinner still going intravenously.

Thurs., Dec. 29/94:
Doing very well. Anticoagulant. Jeffrey visits. Doug told Bev brain surgery.

Fri., Dec. 30/94:
Tried to get out of bed Thursday night [bowel movement]. *Can eat potatoes and meat. Neck brace still on. Will examine neck x-ray. Vici* [Doug's sister] *visits for a few days.*

Sat., Dec. 31/94:
Vici and Doug dry wash Bev's hair while she sat in chair. Got bathed and powdered. After dinner she had ice cream. Leg still swollen. Neck brace still on until doctor OK's to have it taken off.

Sun., Jan. 1/95:
Neck collar off.

Mon., Jan. 2/95:
Had hair washed 3:00 a.m. Doing well. Neck brace off.

Tues., Jan. 3/95:
Beverley phones us 8:15 p.m., talked until 8:30. Voice very weak and low, but cheerful to hear.

Wed., Jan. 4/95:

Therapy? IV out of chest, into arm. Therapy for leg, but not too much…

My stay in Critical Care marked the beginning of an awareness of my situation and condition. I began to remember things that were happening, converse with visitors, move around a little, feel my limitations, experience morphine hallucinations, become frustrated in my discomfort, and be stopped by pain and exhaustion.

I remember trying to eat with my neck in a brace. Unable to tip my head forward or backward, eating was a disaster. A myriad of food items slipped from my fork or spoon onto my chin, and oozed under my neck brace. After a few days my sticky neck reeked of oatmeal.

I remember having to go to the bathroom really, really badly. So inspired, somehow I got up and squeezed between the bed rails, but as soon as my legs touched ground, my now steel rod-reinforced broken leg exploded with so much pain my bowels emptied on the spot. The nurse came running, chastising me for getting up, and warning me to never do that again. Later I remember hearing the roar of the wet vac and smelling the strong odour of disinfectant spray as wayward droplets splashed my face.

Throughout all this I kept my sense of humour and boundless curiosity about what was happening to me and around me.

My outlook was good; in six months I'd be back at work, I thought. But I was in denial. I didn't know then that I wouldn't be able to return to employment. As the months unfolded it slowly became apparent to me that I wasn't the same person I used to be, and my expectations, while still hopeful and at times lofty, would have to be lowered.

My stay in Critical Care was also the start of a very long physical, cognitive, and emotional road to recovery. As I write this, it is almost three years later, and I'm having ongoing problems at all levels. I'm still undergoing physical rehabilitation and am seeing a clinical psychologist every three to four weeks. My emotions are on a roller-coaster ride, as I laugh hysterically one moment and sob the next. There is a lot of fear, anger, depression, sorrow, and frustration; yet, I am aware of how lucky I am when I look at others whom I consider worse off than I—those more physically or cognitively injured. At the same time I feel I have enough to deal with, and it is taking everything I have to cope and stay positive. This leads me to conclude that everything is relative. We are dealt certain cards in life and we have to make the best of them.

Big upheavals always bring long periods of adjustment. My adjustment period continues. Sometimes in my darker hours, I tearfully plead, "Will the real Beverley Richmond please come back?" She's not coming back, I know, but perhaps I can create a Beverley Richmond who will be all right in the long run.

❧ Hallucinations

They say I was a difficult patient. The reality of it was, I was in the 7th floor Neurology Critical Care Unit, drugged on morphine, slipping in and out of consciousness. The first hallucination was that I was in the basement of a warehouse.

"Get me to the hospital," I yelled as I fought against the restraints that secured me in bed. "This isn't a hospital, this is a storage room. Get me to a hospital!"

They say I was argumentative. But wouldn't you be if you thought you were in a basement stockroom of a warehouse somewhere, instead of in a hospital? It was a life and death situation, couldn't they see? And all they did was try to convince me I was in a hospital… and laugh. Under the circumstances, what else could they do?

Another hallucination involved gold jewellery. In it, I just *had* to buy gold jewellery. I went to shop after shop, up and down the main street, visiting all the jewellers in my downtown sales territory, not doing my job selling newspaper ads, but rather—in this hallucination—buying gold jewellery. And I just had to buy it, because you see, it *would get me out of there*. Why, they were holding me against my will for ransom! I even instructed Doug to bring in my own jewellery from home, so we could bribe them into letting me go.

Then I thought I was in a health club. My hallucinations involved hearing the rhythmical pounding of feet in an aerobics class; or, I'd be waiting impatiently for the doors to open or for the instructor to show up for class. There were both men and women in this club, their attire of some interest to me. Men in bikini thongs, for heaven's sake. (Where did *that* come from?)

For two days I insisted I was in a health club, and all Doug could do was humour me. Trying to convince me otherwise was fruitless. (One year later I learned one of my nurses had been a part-time aerobics instructor, and I must have overheard some conversations she'd had with another nurse. Funny how the mind picks up pieces of information and tries somehow to make sense of it all.)

Another hallucination involved having to collect antique German Christmas tree ornaments, and again I searched relentlessly up and down the main street of town for them; I needed enough you see, in order *to get out.* I just had to have them. Working to Christmas deadline, I was. What would happen if I didn't have enough ornaments? They wouldn't let me go! Or would they? How can you be sure when you're hallucinating?

They have a name for this common phenomenon—ICU psychosis. The cause is, (1) confinement; (2) trauma; and (3) definitely, good drugs.

Even later, when I was a little more stabilized and had more wits about me, I was still hallucinatory/hysterical. A blood oxygen monitor is a clip that attaches to the end of a finger or a toe to measure how oxygenated your blood is. It is not a vital monitor, but a helpful one. One day the nurse walked in and nonchalantly removed this monitor from my finger, because she needed it for another patient.

"Bring that back!" I yelled. And yell I did, for a long time, demanding she bring back the monitor because, "I'll die if I don't have it. It's the most important thing, you know," I sobbed. Of course, it wasn't the most important thing, and I wouldn't die without it. Doug and the nurse had a good laugh. In retrospect, it seemed they laughed a lot at me.

Almost eighteen months later I had to undergo a second set of surgeries. As I was wheeled back to my room from the OR following surgery, I'm told I kept mumbling, "It's too dark for the nurses in here." They thought that was funny too—the sun was beaming in on me through the window.

My favourite hallucination of all, which makes Doug laugh to this day, is when he remembers me lying on the hospital gurney, drugged and just out of surgery, shaking my head from side to side in disappointment, sighing and saying, "I can't attend the seminar for cranial reconstruction."

All in all, my early days post-accident were filled with disjointed hallucinations and imaginings. A very insistent, difficult patient, yes, but one who, injured, trapped, and confused, tried to make sense of it all in an effort of self-preservation.

A strong survival instinct lashing out in a fog of half reality. The fight or flight instincts run rampant, fuelled by painkillers and a traumatized brain.

Amusing only in retrospect.

❧ Hospital "Ladies"

After my emergence from seven days in Intensive Care and relocation to Critical Care, I became aware of a steady stream of people to my bedside. Names and faces all intermingled at that point, as I endured ten days of poking and prodding, questions and sensations.

Then I went to "the floor." This is where the comings and goings of the Hospital Ladies began to formally shape my timeless days.

To those uninitiated—you future first-timers—here's

what you might expect in a normal hospital day. I have left out the visits of surgeons, staff doctors, interns, therapists, social workers, family doctors, minister, etc., as well as some of the nurses' visits.

All these "ladies" will visit you in approximately this order: menu lady, towel lady, blood lady, basin lady, pill lady, food lady, tray lady, cleaning lady, juice lady, mail lady, temperature/blood pressure lady, pill lady, food lady, tray lady, library cart lady, juice lady, bed change lady, menu lady, food lady, tray lady, pill lady, tuck-shop lady, juice lady, basin lady, night lady.

Although this list may have already exhausted you, here's an in-depth look at these Hospital Ladies.

Towel lady: Comes first thing in the morning, often before you've opened your eyes. Very fleeting. A glimpse is rare. Leaves a towel and washcloth at the foot of your bed.

Blood Lady: Comes jiggling with test tubes. Often cheery. Best when you are still groggy. Always says thank you.

Basin Lady: Gives you tepid water. Ask for hot. Be nice to this lady. She will wash your back; also, other hard to reach places.

Pill Lady: Stands in doorway. Has keys. Counts a lot. Keeps a list. Don't interrupt while she's counting. Often tells you what you're getting. She knows what you've got. Gives you cold water.

Food Lady: Always working to deadline. Wears funny hat. Doesn't chit chat. Noisy. Claims no responsibility for food quality. Often puts food tray in unreachable places.

Tray Lady: Comes about thirty minutes after Food Lady. Also wears funny hat. Doesn't chit chat either. Is always rushing. Don't know why—meals are eaten already and what's leftover on trays is cold.

Cleaning Lady: A social butterfly. Smiles a lot. Picks up things you've dropped. Changes garbage bags. Cleans toilets. Definitely deserves a raise.

Juice Lady: Also rattles a lot and has a cart. Not a huge selection. Apple and prune juice big hits. Also does ice water.

Mail Lady: Vibrant. Always brings good news. Comes not nearly often enough.

Temperature/Pulse/Blood Pressure Lady: Jiggles less than Blood Lady. Otherwise, very similar. Keeps a list like Pill Lady. A hands-on person.

Library Cart Lady: Very friendly with silver hair. Moves slowly. Knows her inventory.

Bed Change Lady: Sometimes more than one visit per day. Very disturbing. Always readjusts your pillows. Recall occasionally needed to fine-tune height or pitch of bed. Friendly, yet industrious.

Menu Lady: Often unseen. May drop off or pick up menu. Mark what you want to eat sometime in the near future. Would be easier deciding if you could count on a bowel movement sometime in the near future. Order extra crackers for when the prune juice lady comes.

Tuck Shop Lady: Also jiggles and has a cart. Much like home shopping. Carries treasures such as hand lotion, hair conditioner, playing cards. Your link to the real world. Unfortunately, always wants money. Unfortunately, your money always in toe of sock, in bottom drawer, behind supply of three-ply toilet paper from home.

Night Duty Ladies: Travel in groups in darkness. Usually whispering. Most elusive of all the Ladies. Carry a bright light which they shine in your eyes. With any luck, your eyes are closed.

Bless them all.

∾ Visitors

My first visitor was Doug.

Drugged on morphine and wired to life sustaining equipment, I lay in Intensive Care begging, "Help me! You have to help me."

Doug sat stroking my hand, and with tears in his eyes replied helplessly, "I can't."

Highly agitated I cried, "Then don't touch me!"

While these were not my first remembrances of a visitor, they are nonetheless Doug's painful recollection of his first visit following my emergence from the operating room. Yes, I was a grouchy patient then. And why not? Only hours before I had been hit by a van.

My first recollections of visitors are fuzzy. Whether it was in Intensive Care or early days in Critical Care, I remember featureless faces being thrust close to mine. Muffled voices spoke unremembered words, as I was either kissed or stroked on the cheek, my hand squeezed or held. I have only a vague remembrance of who was there, and can only guess at approximately which day.

To me, drifting in and out of awareness, it seemed they had all arrived on one day, all in a row, one after another. A ludicrous assumption, as if there was a line-up waiting to view me. I say "view me," because I was bandaged from head to toe with only my face and hands exposed. All I could do was lie motionless, expressionless.

Later, as awareness and responsiveness increased, my memories became more vivid. Dear friends, family, and acquaintances had travelled to visit—some by train or bus, others by car—from Toronto, Belleville, or the Ottawa area. Some visitors were shy and calm, while others were wildly exuberant. One thing all my visitors had in common was they quickly tired me out.

Some of the more interesting visits included: a co-worker, who got past nurses by masquerading as my brother; a group visit from my advertising buddies at the paper; a dear friend who, knowing my fondness for tea, arrived with a tea party, complete with china cups and saucers, china teapot, and homemade goodies; the head of the downtown business association, who brought well-wishes from all the downtown clients in my sales territory; and my sister-in-law, who came equipped with brush, comb, and hair detangler for my first comb-out approximately ten days following surgery.

Two advertising consultants made a surprise visit to reminisce about a trick they played on me one night after five o'clock at work. One had pretended to be an irate Chinese restaurant owner who complained he had a "beeg boofay, lots of food, but no peepo" (translation: big buffet, lots of food, but no people), and demanded to know where his full-page ad was.

Ironically, I had called on that business earlier in the week and they had placed a small ad. This is what made it so believable—that and the accent. But, I had spoken to a Peter Tom, not his imaginary brother, "Tom Dong" as the caller falsely identified himself. Totally convinced this was a legitimate call and that I had really screwed up, the conversation went on and on until I finally caught on. Did I laugh! What a great prank.

And the joke continued, as unknown to me the whole conversation had been taped. The next morning before I arrived at work, it had been replayed for the editorial department, composing room, and all advertising staff—including my boss. Yes, I had been extremely naive to be fooled like that, but on the plus side I got rave reviews for handling the "irate customer" with kid gloves. Reliving the prank with my visitors and Doug was hilarious therapy.

My dear friends, Barry and Carolyn, visited with a flurry. Possessing an ability to make me laugh at almost anything, they were a joy. As they left, Carolyn scribbled a note on the nurses' blackboard hanging on the wall across from my bed, "You gotta get outta this place!" I agreed.

Another special visit was by my two beautiful sight-hounds. In order to get them into the hospital on therapy dog day, a well-meaning relative created two fake Therapy Dog certificates. This got them into the Rehab ward. Overwhelmed by the unusual sights and smells, the re-enactment of the classic Lassie Come Home reunion I had anticipated didn't materialize. To them, I was the least interesting thing in the room. However, it was still a joy to see and touch them once again after two months' separation.

By the way, their visit helped more than only me. Doug made several stops along the corridor, as other wheelchair-bound patients petted and praised these two well-mannered hounds. The passing-by of the official therapy dogs caused a brief tense moment, but all in all the visit was a success and very comforting. A little bit of love from home.

Visitors are your vital link to the outside world. They are your lifelines to such things as pizza, burgers, ice cream sundaes, your favourite magazines, family photographs, and more. Just seeing them helps you tremendously, but when they can bring you something you need or want they're a bonus. Use them; they want to help, and the opportunity to do so makes them feel needed and of service.

∾

When you're in the hospital you're in a foreign place—an artificial environment—where medical and support staff come and go on their rounds at the prescribed hour. When you add up all their visits, there is a lot of people-contact for the bed-bound patient. But much of this I compare to background music in an office or home, perhaps a radio or TV turned on just for noise.

Real interaction, real company, is best provided by visitors at the patient's bedside. Visitors provide a comforting contact with your normal life—the one you left behind once you passed through those hospital doors. They provide gossip, memories, support, laughs, and love. Although many of the hospital personnel are supportive, helpful, and kind, they can't remind you of home.

Share yourself with someone you know or love who's sick. Visit them in the hospital and, if they're in for an extended period of time, try to visit them on a regular basis. Believe me, it is better to make surprise visits when you are able, than to promise to visit next Tuesday but then never show up. A visitor is a wonderful thing; a visit forgotten is not.

I was blessed with lovely visits from concerned friends and family. I hope you are, too. But if you're not, here's some advice: why don't you give *them* a call? If you can't dial on your own, ask a nurse, aide, or your roommate to dial for you. Hearing their voices will help dissipate that twinge of loneliness you may be feeling. And do you want to know a secret? The patient in the next bed won't mind it if you share his or her visitors, by joining in their conversation just a little now and then.

∾ Hemorrhoids and Other Matters

The two "H" words—hospitals and hemorrhoids. To me they're synonymous.

There's something about hospitals—no doubt the changed menu, inactivity, and resulting irregularity, codeine painkillers, and difficult logistics of just getting to the pot—that promoted good, healthy hemorrhoids in me.

While in Critical Care shortly following my accident, my bowels were fairly regular and using the facilities was mostly painless. First, I'd buzz for the nurse. "I have to go to the bathroom," I'd announce. She'd arrive with a commode (toilet on wheels) and help me onto it. This was difficult; I had a broken right leg, my broken right arm was in a cast, I was weak, and I was hooked up to IV transfusion needles, heart monitors, etc. A curtain was then pulled around the hospital bed area to afford me some measure of privacy. This was effective visually, but not so for the auditory component. However, by careful self-monitoring of bodily excretions and evacuations, I was able to maintain a level of restraint and dignity. When done, I would ring the buzzer to resummon the nurse to assist me back into bed.

I slowly graduated to getting on and off the commode on my own, so I would only have to ring for the nurses to fetch the commode, and then ring for them to remove it. This latter part developed into a problem. For some reason, while nurses speedily brought the commode, they were not so quick to remove it. Lying beside a steaming pot of unmentionables while waiting for the nurse to reappear is a true character builder. "I'm finished," I'd yell into the intercom to hopefully summon assistance sooner.

The next step came when I could be rolled to the actual washroom. The procedure was quite the same. I'd summon the nurse. She'd arrive with a false commode—seat only, no bowl—and roll me into the washroom, positioning me carefully over the toilet bowl, being careful to line me up just right. When done, I'd press the buzzer to summon the nurse, who'd arrive eventually to wheel me back to my bed.

The only problem with this system was the "false security" the commode with no bowl gave me. Once seated on the commode, my body told me, "OK now, let's go," but my mind shouted, "Stop, it's just a chair—there's no bowl under me!" There were some pretty anxious moments but no accidents.

Later on, I could propel myself via wheelchair to the washroom and transfer on and off the toilet myself. What freedom and independence! I was now potty trained. The only problem with this system was that I was not able to (or allowed to) flush. Not able to, because my balance was off and the handle hard to reach. Not allowed to, because the nurses would want to have a look first. (They had been spying at the results all along. Even more unbelievable, they were quantifying them in the earliest days after the accident. Apparently, nurses do this sort of thing.) A healthy stool is a healthy patient.

The next phase was my ability to not only maneuver to and from and on and off the toilet, but also to flush. Little did I suspect that flushing the evidence would elicit a new form of "intelligence." "Did your bowels move?" became the question of the day. A "yes," or "no" was not sufficient enough a reply. Rather, gradations were required: "small," "medium," or "large."

But after a while, there were days when there was no movement. Then days in a row with no movement. So, next came "stool softener" pills and laxatives, but these had no effect. At this point I should have lied about the lack of results, for unwittingly I was setting myself up for the feared suppositories. These came in all sizes and strengths. Some elicited mediocre response, others no response. Soon I was begging for help. "You and your bowels!" one frustrated nurse exclaimed. It seemed to me something else was wrong. I would sit and sit, but nothing would happen, although I would feel I had accomplished a lot. I had hemorrhoids blocking the pathway, so no amount of suppository dynamite or enemas would help.

In the meantime my stay in the Rehab Unit was coming to an end, and discharge day from the hospital came and went. With the increased activity at home, increased appetite, and more food options, my bowels moved ever so slightly.

At a routine GP appointment following my release, I asked doctor Andy to check me out. I bared all. An astonished silence broke as he exclaimed, "That's a big one!"

Armed with pills, hemorrhoid creams, bulk stool

softeners, and orders to drink lots of water, I left his office. My regimen began.

Slowly, things improved. One by one the arsenal decreased, as healthy regularity returned to my digestive tract.

ଏ

Constipation and hemorrhoids are a common problem for the long-term hospital patient. What can be learned from my experience? Some painkillers paralyze the bowels. For me, codeine did that, so for future stays in the hospital I said I was allergic to codeine, so that morphine, Demerol, or extra-strength Tylenol (not Tylenol III which contains codeine) were prescribed instead for pain.

Inactivity is the other culprit for inducing constipation and hemorrhoids. For this reason, after my subsequent surgeries Doug had me up and walking laps around the hospital corridors to help keep my muscle tone (abdominal and elsewhere) from atrophy. Gentle abdominal massages also helped keep things moving.

Getting regular exercise and eating a varied diet of fruits and vegetables daily, bran cereal, avoiding seeds, nuts, spicy food, garlic, and chocolate, plus drinking lots of water, help keep me, now, for the most part, hemorrhoid trouble-free.

ଏ The Dining Room

"Will you be eating in your room or in the dining room?" the nurse asks.

"The dining room?"

"Yes, there's a dining room where many patients like to eat their meals. Would you like to go and socialize?"

I ponder the question.

"No," I respond, "I'll eat at the side of my bed again, thank you."

This is the second month of hospitalization in the Rehab Ward, and I'm wheelchair bound. I look terrible, feel terrible, and certainly don't want to "socialize" with other patients.

Days go by and the same question is asked again and again at mealtimes. And each time the nurses seem disappointed with my decision.

Finally, I give in. "I'll give it a try," I say.

So, off I go, wheeled to the other end of the floor. I enter the crowded dining room—three long tables lined on both sides with wheelchairs. It's a tight fit, but I'm in.

Being "the new one" I'm somewhat of an oddity. I smile at the questioning and sometimes vacant faces around me as I'm handed a large bib.

The food trays arrive in a flurry of nurses, special meals going to special patients, each tray as ordered by each patient, days before, from a multiple-choice menu left at bedside. Surrounded by grey hair, I watch as feeble eyes and uncooperative hands fumble with milk cartons, sugar packets, soup lids, single wrapped portions of salad dressing, butter and such.

Before too long I'm helping, and have appointed myself "nurses' assistant in charge of opening" at the table. The wrinkled smiles express their thanks as cartons, lids, straws, and packets are opened, and joyful dining begins.

The talk is sparse, as eating is serious work and requires complete concentration from everyone. Nevertheless, food escapes to laps, bibs, faces, hands, and the floor all around me.

A TV perches in the corner of the dining room, and there is an aerobics instructor on the screen demonstrating geriatric exercises. She says, "Age is a state of mind. If you don't mind, you won't age." Strangely, this strikes me as funny and I laugh out loud. Looking around, I notice I am the only one laughing.

The nurses are busy again, for as quickly as the food-laden trays arrived, now emptied, they begin to disappear. With them go the patients. There is a traffic jam as nurses and patients entangle with other wheelchairs in the rush back to the rooms. Why are they rushing, I wonder?

I sit until the last is wheeled out.

From then on I eat in the dining room from time to time only. Although the dining room is a distracting change, my weakened emotional and mental state cannot handle the reality of it. Most of the diners are aged female stroke victims, a too vivid reminder of the fate awaiting many women, including, perhaps, myself.

I feel badly, guilty too, that my thoughts betray within me the existence of a hierarchy of sickness—a prejudice of incapacity. Yes, I was almost killed in a traffic accident, but I'm not *that* bad off.

I am embarrassed by my thoughts.

✍ Menopause or MVA? (Motor Vehicle Accident)

The article read, "Overall Symptoms—headaches, hot flashes, insomnia, sweating, dizziness, anxiety, depression, irritability, loss of concentration, changes in sex drive, incontinence, vaginal dryness, bone aches and pains."

I looked up from the article and stared in wonderment. The newspaper dropped from my hands. Except for "incontinence" and "vaginal dryness" I had all the symptoms.

The revelation hit me as if I had been struck on the head with a bedpan. "My God!" I laughed. "I didn't get hit, thrown, and run over by a van (MVA: Motor Vehicle Accident); I had menopause at the corner of Front and Victoria!"

While in the hospital I appreciated any bit of humour, even though sometimes it was preposterous and self-directed purposefully to poke fun at my predicament. For days I had a lot of fun showing the article to friends and family, relating such an outrageous notion.

Speaking of menopause, my period stopped for three months following the accident. The trauma, the shock to my system, temporarily delayed it. Not a bad tactic for Mother Nature to take when faced with the question, "Can this body nourish and protect a growing new life, while all its energy is focused on keeping itself, the bodily host, alive? No."

Tied into this was my low hospital body weight—a mere 89 pounds. Apparently, an adult female at 85 pounds is in danger of halting menstruation, a problem seen in young gymnasts, and I was very close to that weight.

My abdomen had been bloated for quite some time, with much tenderness and some pain on both sides. I was complaining daily to the doctor and nurses, but they were unsure as to what was wrong. You see, I was also very constipated— the thinking was, this was the reason for my discomfort.

But then it finally started. I remember the night.

In a heady wave of excitement, I searched for the cord to summon the nurse. Pressing the buzzer, I shouted triumphantly, "I've got my period! Bring me a pad!"

The response was deadpan, "Oh yeah, I'll bring the champagne, too."

Shortly afterward, two nurses appeared; one handed me a big brown paper bag. Quizzically, I opened the bag and unwrapped its contents; there was one extra-huge, superduper, queen-size incontinence pad. I stared at it with startled surprise on my face, then collapsed back into bed in uncontrollable laughter.

The laughter was contagious. Both nurses burst, and the sound of our hysterics brought other nurses running to share in the fun.

A great prank. That laughter was the best, pure, sweet medicine.

ᕦ Interesting People

If you're in the hospital now, take a moment to look around you—there are interesting people everywhere.

One early evening my hospital roommate and I were startled by an elderly man standing in the doorway in his pajamas, or rather, in his pajama tops. Pajama bottoms missing. Bottoms up. Helpless in our beds, roommate Bonnie turns and whispers across the darkened room to me, "I've got a knife!" flashing a small, plastic dinner knife menacingly in his direction. The stranger in our doorway stands there, shifting from foot to foot, mumbling something at us, staring in our direction. We listen, caught in suspended animation. Shortly, a nurse quietly appears, takes our intruder gently by the arm, and escorts him away.

One evening Doug and I headed for the daytime dining room, come evening TV-room, for a change of scenery. He wheels me in, we hang a left turn, and park. Once settled we glance behind us to the other side of the room at some people there. Seated in a wheelchair, an elderly male patient is receiving a nose hair trimming executed carefully by a uniformed attendant. No words are exchanged between them. In the quiet of the room, the methodical snipping is mesmerizing. Doug and I gaze upon this sight momentarily, smile discreetly at each other, then leave the room and this seemingly secretive ritual.

This interesting guy is a young neurosurgeon. He walks in one day and asks me why I'm on blood thinners. Startled, I look at him and respond, "Because I have mechanical heart valves."

"No you don't," he says.

"Yes I do," I say, dumbfounded by his response.

"They're not on the x-rays," he explains.

"Well, I have them," I respond, pulling out two wallet cards which clearly show the serial number and model number of the valves, one card for each mechanical heart valve, the date installed in me, and the surgeon's name. That should prove it, I think.

He studies the cards. "Well, I can't see them."

I take this as a personal challenge. When he leaves the room, I phone St. Jude Medical Inc. in Minnesota, the manufacturer of the valves, and ask. I learn the valves are made of a specialized coated-carbon, pyrolytic carbon, and have a polyester sewing cuff. They sometimes don't show up on x-rays due to their positioning within the heart. I relay the information to the surgeon. If you don't believe me, check my hospital file, I think.

Days later I receive in the mail from St. Jude two samples of actual heart valves, plus some literature and writing pads complete with heart motif. The valves make a great show-and-tell; the nurses and surgeon are fascinated. It finally hits me that, after all, this is the neuroscience ward, not the cardiology ward, so what would a young brain surgeon know about heart valves?

This next interesting guy, you hear long before you see him. The closer he gets, the less you want him in your room. A loud distraction, yes, but he's the guy that picks up things from far under the bed which you dropped there days ago.

The vacuum man appears, his shiny, black hair slicked back into a long ponytail, his five o'clock shadow closer to 6:30. Odd looking, for a fifty-plus-year-old hospital worker, I puzzle.

In he roars, moving back and forth, back and forth, back and forth, concentrating on his work. Shutting off the machine, he stops to retrieve the spoon from under my bed. Now is my chance to interact with this unusual character.

"Thanks!" I say as he hands me the spoon. As our conversation unfolds, it turns out this mild-mannered hospital worker drove a "hog" for twenty years, the 1000 cc's of vibrating Harley Davidson now replaced by the roar of a hospital vacuum cleaner.

Definitely interesting people.

❧

There are lots of people all around you at the hospital. Since you're laid up there for a while anyway, why not take some time to stop, look, and wonder. I guarantee it will help make the strange journey you're on a little more enjoyable and, well, interesting.

∾ The Weekend Pass

There came a time, after about eight weeks in the hospital, when I had improved to the point of being able to transfer in and out of a wheelchair, as well as propel and maneuver myself for short distances, that I was offered the option of a "weekend pass."

I hadn't heard of such a practice before, so naturally the idea seemed odd at first. The rehab doctor explained that a weekend pass was a trial release from the hospital, an opportunity to see how it goes, how I fared. It was a practice session, as it were, and part of my rehabilitation.

Knowing about the existence of "the weekend pass" helped explain why the ward was generally quieter with fewer visitors on the weekends. Obviously, many patients took advantage of it and did their entertaining at home.

I, however, didn't want to go. I was scared to leave the hospital and resisted the notion for a couple of weeks, until my husband and the rehabilitation doctor finally convinced me it was time to give it a try. On February 24/95, approximately two months after the accident, I headed home for the weekend.

It seemed too soon for me to attempt a trial stay, because only two days earlier the same rehab doctor had said it would be three to four months before I could put full weight on my right leg. Hearing that had upset, frustrated, and depressed me. I took the information as meaning I'd be hospitalized for another three or four months. That wasn't what he'd meant at all. And so there I was, going home for the weekend. But how?

To help us out, our enterprising neighbour, utilizing resources available, organized a school bus with a handicap wheelchair lift for my journey home. Once the wheelchair and I were strapped into place inside the bus, the ride began. The next-to-nothing shocks and an over-exuberant driver resulted in an awful, but exciting, trip home. When I sighted the house, tears flowed. My beautiful, country, Victorian farmhouse—my home— there it was at last. It was wonderful to return, if only for a short visit.

While getting into the van via the wheelchair lift was fairly straightforward, getting into the house was another matter. The stairs, which loomed in front of us, frightened me. John, our lumberjack of a neighbour, had to tip the wheelchair backward slightly, so his wife and Doug could lift the front up while he pulled the wheelchair up the steps backwards. When he tipped the chair back I instinctively thrust my body forward trying to keep the wheelchair and myself upright. I screamed, "No, I'll fall. My head! I'll fall and hurt my head."

"Relax, you'll be OK. You won't fall. We won't let you," were the comforting replies from the three. I resigned myself to the fact that this might be the end of me, right there and then on my very own doorstep, so I closed my eyes and relaxed. Before I knew it, I was up the stairs, into the house, and plunked in the middle of the kitchen. I gazed around. Everything looked so strange yet familiar; I recalled how my parents' home seemed strange when we returned from my grandfather's cottage at the end of the summer when I was young. I had been hospitalized for three months, much longer than any summer vacation, so the strangeness was to be expected.

Soon a more urgent thought pressed. The bathroom! I had to go to the bathroom. Carefully, I eased myself down the 2″ step from the kitchen into the living room. With this forward momentum and the slope of the old floors, I rolled uncontrollably across the floor and smack into the wall. This bit of slapstick comedy helped ease the tension of the moment. Unhurt, I wheeled to the facilities still laughing.

Home-cooked macaroni and cheese, wieners, spaghetti—these were my menu choices for the weekend. And, boy, did they taste good! My appetite would be best described as ravenous. (At the time I didn't know my weight had shrunk to less than 90 pounds while in the hospital. My body was literally starving.)

During that first weekend home, I passed the time in horizontal mode for the most part; sitting up for any length of time was exhausting. Visitors' stays were kept short. Memories of the two days are few.

By Sunday afternoon I found this weekend pass stuff much too taxing and was glad to head back to the comfort, convenience, and familiarity of my hospital bed in the Rehab Ward. If you had asked me that Sunday evening, I never would have guessed that, the following weekend, I'd consent to go home again on another pass, and that the next weekend I'd be released from hospital.

The weekend pass is a necessary evil of recovery, and a stepping stone for return to the outside world.

∾

There is a real anxiety about weekend passes to the long-term hospital patient. It's a leap into the unknown, in a sense, with fear of failure attached to it. Without the security and support of the familiar hospital regime, we feel like helpless babes.

The first weekend pass home may prove difficult, exhausting, and over-stimulating. It did for me. I think it's that way for everyone. The second weekend pass will be easier for both the patient and the caregiver. And hopefully after that, the patient will be well enough, and confident enough, to leave hospital permanently.

∾ Others' Reactions

It's impossible to do a thorough job detailing all the reactions of those who also experienced my accident. Some cannot, to this day, talk about it. Others are no longer around to talk about it. Many cannot remember anything in particular, except that they were shocked and upset when they heard about it.

Somehow, not knowing how customers, co-workers, friends, and relatives reacted leaves a void—the void of not knowing how I impacted on people. Perhaps I feel there's some sort of a rating system—the more you react, the more you care. And this is probably true to much extent. Why it matters to me is more the question.

Maybe it simply mattered to know how much they

cared for me. Maybe deep inside I wanted to know how much I'd wrecked their day, for surely this would be an indication of how much I impacted on them? I'm sorry and enraged the accident happened, but I also feel guilty upsetting, hurting, inconveniencing, and disappointing so many people—especially as it happened four days before Christmas. Odd thought, for someone who has suffered so much, isn't it? Why should I care about how hurt they were, for heaven's sake; I'm the one that suffered the near-fatal injuries. I cared because I loved them.

Maybe I'm wondering about "reactions" because the accident was the most significant, intense, exciting event in my life, yet I remember hardly anything about it. I know the pain of it all is embedded deep inside me, but I'm missing what went on around me, to the people around me. What did they experience? What did they see? What did they hear? What did they feel?

Asking someone how he reacted to my accident is a little like saying, "Since I'm really important in your life, you'll remember with clarity the details of every minute following my near-fatal episode, right? Tell me, how did you feel?" This just can't be done. When I did ask a fellow co-worker, seven months post-accident, about what he remembered of that day, he responded, "Well, it's not like it was the assassination of JFK, you know." Well, so much for that topic of conversation.

For relatives, it's too painful. For my husband, it's reliving his worst nightmare. Why do it? To satisfy my curiosity or ease my feelings of insecurity? Not good enough.

So, buried it remains. More missing pieces of the jigsaw puzzle that is my accident.

Nevertheless, there is one reaction I shall always remember.

Several months after the accident I longed for Chinese food, so we made an outing to our favourite local haunt in the County. As we entered the restaurant, the owner looked up at me and excitedly asked, "Where have you been? Haven't seen you in soooo long."

"I got hit and run over by a van," I replied matter-of-factly.

After a moment's pause she exclaimed, "Don't doooo that!" I just laughed.

❧ Cards and Letters

My stay in Intensive Care involved no recollection of cards and letters. What minute recollections I did have were either drug-induced hallucinations or mere fragments of events rising out of a fog of timelessness.

My stay in Critical Care involved the beginning of visits by family and friends, and the knowledge that some people had called with well wishes. It wasn't until I moved out of Critical Care to "the floor" that the deluge began.

Oh, how I was surprised each day when the mail lady brought a handful of cards. Each card meant as much to me as any Christmas gift. And the variety of cards—the funny ones, the sincere ones, the inspirational ones, the beautiful ones, the corny ones, and the card with the bouquet of purple lilacs on the cover that brought a flood of tears to my eyes.

Lilacs meant so much to me. They reminded me of my country home on a lilac-lined lane—a home which I would, despite bad odds, see again soon. And what a heavenly smell there would be. Lilacs—the promise of spring, my favourite time of the year—epitomize the glorious colour and beauty of nature. All this emotion from one little card.

Another favourite was the card with the bowl of chunky chicken noodle soup on the cover, which read inside, "The chicken feels worse," so articulating my present state of mind and body that I burst into laughter.

Each greeting meant the sender had taken time out of their busy schedule to think about me, seek out a card, and send it on its way. I was in their thoughts and their prayers. How lovely.

The cards piled up, and each night when my husband visited I eagerly showed him the cards and delivered full explanations about who the senders were. I must admit that, at times, I felt a bit spoiled and embarrassed—I had a pile of cards, while the elderly lady in the next bed had only a few. She particularly liked the card with a picture of a puppy on the front, whose big plastic eyes moved in circles when the card was shaken. She told me she had once had a dog named Blackie, whom she said, "loved more and had a better heart" than many people she'd known. Touched by her story, I gave her the card to keep by her bedside. With tearful eyes, she accepted it gratefully. When her son arrived to visit that evening it was a topic of pleasant conversation for them to share.

Not only did the cards keep coming, but oh, the plants and flowers. And like the cards, they came in all shapes and sizes, all colours and aromas. The fragrance upon entering my hospital room was heavenly. What interest and comments they generated, too.

Fortunately, the time soon came for me to transfer to another hospital closer to home, but with that also came the frigid January transfer of my plants. Two befell an amusing fate.

My transporter, who shall remain nameless, was exiting the down elevator with an armful of my plants, when a man entered the elevator on his way up. "I'll give you $25 for those two plants," the man said. A second's hesitation by my transporter ended with "Okay!" When he returned to pick up the next batch of plants, he informed me my plants had not only made me some money, they had also made another patient in the hospital very happy. I was a bit angry—after all he had sold two of my most beautiful plants—but I was even more amused at the lunacy of the situation, as well as satisfied the new owner would probably be as thrilled with the plants as I had been. On another day, when he was offered money in the elevator for the pizza he was taking up for us to share, he flatly refused without any hesitation. Everyone has priorities.

Nevertheless, most of the Kingston plants successfully made it to Belleville. My immobility, the dry hospital air, and the busy nurses all conspired the discard of many potted plants that hadn't been regularly watered. Cut flowers were all the more appreciated in this hot environment, but still some fared better than others. The breathtaking beauty of the dozen long-stemmed roses was far too short-lived; it seems roses "don't do well" in hospitals. Mine were recycled when one of the nurses spotted the crispy, darkened flowers in the garbage bin and joyfully claimed them for use in a floral wreath she was creating at home.

After arriving home at last, the remaining hyacinth and crocus bulbs were eventually replanted in my garden, as were the chrysanthemums. A small houseplant, which a co-worker presented me in the hospital, survived in my home as a beautiful memory of him for almost two years following his sudden death.

Two of my most wonderful cards were the "group" cards—one from my office buddies at *The Intelligencer,* and one from the downtown merchants in my sales territory. Each card contained a myriad of signatures. Voluptuous cards they were, filled with greetings and comments from friends and clients. Those cards were especially important to me.

Of course, after I left the hospital three months later, the cards came less and less often. So, perhaps one of the sweetest cards I ever received was that lone, single greeting from my friend Elizabeth eight months after the accident, that pictured a tiny, sewn-up teddy bear propped up on the floor in the corner of an empty room, looking and feeling much like me. The card read, "Just when you think you're alone... someone lets you know they're thinking about you!" That one hit the spot and made my day.

I have taken out my collection of cards occasionally and reread them. Each time they make me feel happy, contented, and bring back many fond memories of healthier times.

∾

It is extremely important to keep sending those cards and letters. The first onslaught of generous wishes is appreciated and wonderful, but those little notes and cards that trickle in after many months have passed are guaranteed to help lift the sagging spirit of your, perhaps now neglected, convalescing friend or relative.

Believe me, they will appreciate those tiny messages of love.

✆ Depression, Loneliness, Isolation

To describe the depression I'm feeling five months after the accident is difficult. Where do I start?

There's the depression that arises out of knowing someone has changed your life forever, in one careless moment, and their life appears to continue on much as before. Is it anger or resentment I'm experiencing here? I don't know, but, definitely, they're both contributing factors.

There's the depression of realizing my life will be only what I make of it; that beyond me lies a great challenge. Will I overcome the obvious physical handicaps? Will I survive the upcoming two operations, and will I be better off or worse off after?

There's the depression over the uncertain future. What will become of my career now? Will I recover enough to continue my job in advertising and, if so, will I be as successful, or will my cognitive abilities (or rather non-abilities) interfere, preventing me from being as successful as I once was? Will this lack of achievement eat away at my self-confidence and render me even more depressed over my losses?

If I can't return to my past job, what will I do, and what will become of me? Will I make enough money? To me, work and security are of utmost importance. How will I get by?

How has the accident hurt other parts of my body? What has been changed internally during the trauma and accident? What lies waiting within me to suddenly emerge one day as another level of challenge or adversity to overcome? What if I've lost my will to live; what if I cannot muster the internal strength one more time to pull myself through another medical crisis?

There's the depression over a lost life and fear of the unknown. Who am I now? I'm not the same person I was. I think differently. I act differently. I feel differently. Again I ask, "Who am I? Who will I be five years from now?"

There's depression resulting from the guilt I feel over the increased strain this whole incident has caused my husband, family, and friends; depression over my changed relationship with others; and depression concerning my new high level of self-pity and self-involvement.

When will this end? Just as I think I'm turning the corner and see the ray of hope, that ray of sunshine, the silver lining in the cloud—something happens to send me into another bout of depression. How does one not feel depressed over a lost year? Or over a lost ten days where there is no recollection of anything, save a few drug-induced hallucinations.

There's the depression that loneliness brings. How time heals old wounds. How time erases people from other people's lives. How life goes on. You're there one day, then gone the next. For a while people seek you out, look for you, call you, visit you. Then time steps in, and suddenly they get along quite well without you, thank you very much, and oh, yes, how *are* you doing today?

There's the loneliness of being plucked from a busy,

active life filled with people of all kinds, and left in an isolated (albeit idyllic) setting. Loneliness due to having a
small, geographically scattered family, and a social net-
work revolving around a career that has suddenly ended
and is no longer a possibility. There's the frustration of
being isolated and now dependent on others to get
around; the loss of spontaneity and independence, all contributing further to my depression.

There's the pang of regret for not having been at work
to see a favourite co-worker one last time prior to his sudden death. And there's bewilderment over the loss, again
by sudden death, of the man who placed the blanket over
me that December day as I lay on the frozen road after the
accident. Why didn't I call him on that day (two days
before his death) to say hello and thanks again for being so
kind to visit me in the hospital, something my gut told me
to do but which I ignored, putting off to another day.
Another day which never came in time for me, or for him.

And there's the depression caused by the realization
that I will be depressed for no particular reason other than
depression results from a brain injury.

The key to all this, I suppose, is to accept the depression as a step in my recovery. I'm told it will pass and it's
not something to be embarrassed or self-critical about. So,
I will cry, wail, sob uncontrollably—just let it out—and
perhaps one day the last tears of fear, depression, and
loneliness will be cried.

ॐ

This chapter on depression and loneliness was the first
one written of this book, which I began five months after

the accident. It has been difficult for me. Almost five years later I'm still considered, by the clinical psychologist, depressed. Although antidepressants have been mildly suggested, I've decided against them, choosing natural alternatives and coping strategies. I've accepted the fact I won't be returning to work full time. Often I feel sad about that, however, it has afforded me new opportunities for personal growth and for doing things I didn't have the time for prior to the accident.

Some people have asked what happened to the driver. I don't know, other than the fact she was charged with careless driving. Do you hate her, they want to know. No, I don't. She didn't intend to hit me—it was an accident. Yes, I'm sorry I got hit, but I'm not angry with her. Since she has not been in contact with me, I can only assume she's having psychological difficulties coping with the guilt arising out of that one careless moment.

As one way of coping, you may find it helpful to get your feelings down in black and white on paper like I did. It's hard to do. I shed lots of tears as I was writing, when sensitive issues were expressed, but found it had a purging effect, somewhat like throwing out the dirty dishwater or taking out the garbage. It's helpful to take some time to reflect upon what you've written, then, at some future date, look back at your notes to see how far you've come.

Reading your thoughts and feelings aloud to someone close to you—a trusted friend, relative, spouse, or therapist, for example—also helps deal with these negative emotions and lets others know what you're going through. Understanding and a little sympathy go a long way.

Remember "peaks and valleys?" "Good times and bad

times?" When you've hit bottom, things can only get better. You have, despite all odds, survived. Take that strength, that will to live which has demonstrated itself so amazingly, and be proud of your achievements. Be thankful. No, go all the way... be happy to be alive. Each and every day *is* a gift, regardless of how that gift comes wrapped. Welcome it, savor it, appreciate it, experience it. Love it. Love yourself. To have survived all this, you deserve that.

"Think of yourself as an accident victim walking away from the crash: your old life has crashed and burned; your new life isn't apparent yet. You may feel yourself to be temporarily without a vehicle. Just keep walking."

—From *The Artist's Way*, by Julia Cameron, on the volatile and changeable shifts of identity

⨀ Excuse Me, May I Please Have the Rest of My Skull Back?

After a three month hospital stay and fourteen months of ongoing rehabilitation following the accident, I was back in May '96 for "cosmetic" elective surgery, as they called it. Putting a 3 x 4 inch piece of skull bone back into my head somehow didn't seem like cosmetic or elective surgery, but that's what the folks at the hospital called it.

There was one snag, however. They couldn't put the same piece of bone back in because, they said, while it was being stored at -70 degrees in the hospital bone bank, it thawed out during a power failure exactly one year and one day after the accident. As a result, they used acrylic bone putty to patch up the hole in my skull.

Due to complications arising from a careless dressing change after the surgery by a harried nurse, and my tendency to bleed, I developed a large hematoma that jeopardized the site. What should have been a one-week stay in the hospital lasted three weeks. I was sent home to heal, but the wound putrefied. In July '96, I returned for more surgery to cut away and remove infected or dead bone, skin, and tissues, to rotate scalp, and to graft skin.

This chapter describes this last surgery and the months following. It is the most detailed chapter and was the most difficult emotionally to write. It relates my soul's dilemma before and after the second scalp surgery. You will witness a supreme struggle of wills involving the question of whether to live or die. You may find some of what you read upsetting—it is not for the queasy or faint of heart.

∞

It's July 1, 1996. Seated at the window of the Sleepless Goat, I watch. On the street an assortment of people walk, ride, cycle, or drive by, some with kids, some with dogs, some alone, some with friends or family. In the restaurant a collection of students and well-dressed seniors dine. How carefree, naturally animated, absorbed, and *healthy* they are, I observe.

In contrast, I sit there with a thick slash of white gauze encircling my head. Neither carefree, nor animated, nor healthy, I am terribly absorbed. It's an absorbing thought to think I am an oddity and a bystander, watching life and the world whiz by as I crawl from one medical moment to another.

Today I am to be admitted to hospital for more surgery. I am not happy about it, but it has to be done. Here we go again, I think; it's beginning to get boring. The novelty is gone, and I'm literally both sick and tired from it all.

At the hospital the routine begins. A nurse does a weigh-in and asks many questions regarding my medical condition, medical history, and current medications. I know it's there already in my file, but I guess they want it all again. My vitals (temperature, blood pressure, and pulse) are checked, as well as a listen to my heart. Doug and I chuckle when our first nurse turns out to be Danielle, one of the nurses who attended me during my stay in Neurosurgery's Critical Care Unit (NCCU) following my accident in December '94. She's glad to see me looking so well this time around. As I look at her, I think about how their jobs lack closure, how they move from one patient to another, one crisis to another, without ever knowing the outcome.

Except in my case.

This is my fifth stay in four years at Kingston General.

The first was in August '92, for open-heart surgery to install artificial aortic and mitral valves.

The second stay came approximately ten days after discharge, when my heart sac ballooned with post-surgery fluid and I was rushed by ambulance to have the fluid surgically removed.

The third visit, in December '94, was for emergency surgery to repair a broken arm, broken leg, fractured skull, and intracerebral bleeding following the accident. The stay lasted one month in the hospital's Neuroscience unit, and continued for two more months in Belleville General Hospital's Rehabilitation unit.

The fourth visit was in May '96, to cover the hole where the surgeons had removed a piece of skull bone in order to relieve pressure due to brain swelling following the accident.

This is now my fifth visit; it is July 1/96, and I have had enough. The acrylic bone patch in my skull is infected, and I'm here to have it removed. I can only guess at my length of stay, but I predict at least two weeks.

Back to my story.

The next visitor, after my check-in, is the senior medical student acting as an admitting clerk. Because he's not using a hospital form but rather a scrap of paper, I suspect his tiresome questions, suspiciously similar to the nurse's questions, are nothing more than raw data for a medical paper, or for today's doctor quiz. This is a teaching hospital, after all.

The routine has begun. It's close to 5:00 p.m., and in comes the food tray lady with my first night's meal. I stare at the tray. A flood of memories return, memories of too many bad days in the hospital and too few good days period.

As I fight back the tears, I lift the lid and gaze at the food. The menu planner checklist for the next few days catches my eyes. Although I am lucky to be in a hospital that offers their patients meal choices, it is the same food, listed in the same order, as last time. That does it.

The tears flow, flooding my eyes. I'm crying now, sitting up in bed crying my eyes out over a simple hospital meal and all it represents. Doug comforts me, reminding me I don't have to eat off the meal tray, that I can eat in either of the two cafeterias, and he will gladly get take-out for me from anywhere. I love this guy. What would I do without him?

It's time for him to leave now, and I miss him already. Armed with my list of things to bring tomorrow, and a job list of things for him to do daily, every other day, and weekly, he turns, picks up my empty suitcase, and goes. Suddenly I feel abandoned, alone, afraid. He'll be back tomorrow, but a lot will happen to me between now and then.

This evening's doctor shows up to explain that my blood will be taken tonight and an IV started. My heart sinks. I'd hoped to have one night of freedom before they hook me up to intravenous; one evening to roam the halls, watch TV, and luxuriate unencumbered in my private hospital room with a bath. A bath. One nice soak in a tub before all hell breaks loose would be nice, but that's not meant to be.

Shortly the nurse arrives rattling with a caddy of tubes and, inflicting minimal pain, takes her various vials for blood work. She'll leave the IV insertion to another, more experienced nurse, she explains, in honour of my rather agitated, apprehensive state. I thank her profusely for her good judgement. The pro arrives and after one unsuccessful attempt, inserts and starts the IV, but still there's pain, discomfort, and tears. I am a wreck, and by now everyone here knows it.

There's the urine sample yet to do, but that's the easy part. The hard part is maneuvering the IV pole, to which I'm attached, in and around the bed, chair, tray, door, toilet, sink, and back again. Soon my tranquilizer (by request) will arrive, and I will sleep.

A good, drug-induced sleep. Marvelous. I awaken at 6:00 a.m. to use the bathroom, and notice a new bandage on my arm. I went to bed with three bandages and awoke with four. Obviously, the blood lady struck again. The next time I awaken it's 7:30 a.m., and that vampire is back for more. She is more familiar to me than anyone, for I've started each morning of past visits with her smiling face and pleasant voice, and regardless of which stay at that hospital, she has been the one constant. Too bad she's out for blood. Now I have five bandages and she is gone.

The rest of the morning brings the usual: breakfast tray; nurse with pills; a nurse's aide to help make a cup of unwanted coffee magically turn into a hot cup of tea; a student doctor; surgeons with student doctors; nurse with towels and a bandage change; a friendly nurse who stops by just to say hello; an orderly to take me to x-ray; the cleaning lady; and soon, lunch.

Lunch is tasty. I gobble down the cream of broccoli soup, spaghetti with meat sauce, whole wheat bread with butter, tea, and a fresh orange. Feeling full and lazy, I fall asleep.

Later in the afternoon Doug arrives brimming with smiles, bearing surprises and goodies and things I asked him to bring from home, such as my tiny travel clock, health journal, herbal teas, etc. He's full of energy and wants to know all about what happened since last night when he left.

The dinner tray comes. The food looks too gassy for me, so off he goes to the cafeteria to fetch a huge bowl of pasta with Alfredo sauce. Two pastas in one day? I'm definitely stockpiling carbs. After walking me four laps around the hospital floor, he leaves. I'm sad to see him go, and I can tell he misses me already. Later that evening he phones to tell me something or other, but I know it's to hear my voice and to say, "I love you."

Shortly afterwards, I learn there's no chance of surgery tomorrow because the OR is full. Since Thursdays are clinic days for the neurosurgeons, the next bet for surgery might be Friday. I call Doug to let him know. It is not good news; I should have waited until tomorrow to tell him. At least I can get something to help *me* sleep tonight.

Wednesday's highlights are a shower and Doug's visit. The neurosurgeon also visits to let me know he'll try to coordinate surgery for Friday. He has to coordinate with the plastic surgeon from a nearby hospital to assist with the closure of my skin. The neurosurgeon will open my head to remove the bone patch and infected tissues; the plastic surgeon will close by rotating scalp and skin around to, hopefully, make me like new. This is ridiculous, because I'll have a bald area, scars, and a skull-less depression on the right side of my head.

Wondering about my meals today? Nondescript. I eat what I like and leave the rest. The real highlight of the day is a Therapeutic Touch session administered by one of the nurses.

Being in a highly agitated state and having read about the procedure recently, I decided to ask if Therapeutic Touch was available to patients. The nurse made some inquiries and sent another nurse—my nurse Monika from the Critical Care Unit over a year ago—to my bedside during her scheduled break.

She performed her craft as I lay there, her hands hovering and circling, whisking and flicking over and through the energy current a few inches from my body. To describe the sensation, I would say it's like experiencing the feeling of wavy heat rising off a boiling hot tarmac. You know how the air currents seem to ripple and wave? That's how my body felt as her hands glided skillfully above me. Afterward I felt extreme relaxation as well as increased sensation and circulation to the afflicted side of my head. I elected to lie very, very still for a while after to savor that calm feeling, then fell into a restful afternoon sleep.

Things go smoothly until Thursday morning when the neurosurgeon drops the bombshell: Friday's surgery is off, and I won't be operated on until the following Wednesday when the plastic surgeon from the other hospital will be able to assist. When he leaves, I fall apart.

(In actuality, here is where I stopped writing this chapter using the "write as it happens" method. The news of another delay in surgery plunged me into a psychological and emotional nosedive. It is now nineteen months later as I resume writing. From what I remember, next came a battle between the will to live and a strong desire to give up. My memory fails me [such is the nature of brain injury], but my hospital journal comes to the rescue.)

I cry a lot today. Somehow, all manner of help in the form of visitors is drawn to me, all types of caring people who love me magically come to my aid—nurses, my rehabilitation manager, my friend Rae, Doug, phone calls from my brothers, sister-in-law, sister Barb, and my physiother-apist. Palliative Care arranges for a loaner of a VCR and video, and Doug joins me on the bed to cuddle through the film. Comforting, nice. A day of support and love.

In the meantime, there is increased drainage from my rotting skull and scalp; it's greeny-brown in colour, less red, and I can feel this drainage flowing inside my head at the back of my throat behind my ear. There's far more pus, white blood cells, and bacteria than 4500 mg. of penicillin a day can control.

Today I am lucky to get outside for a while onto the patio in front of the hospital. The sun, breeze, and chirping birds are a lovely break. Those things always affect me positively—appreciating and revering nature is my great-est source of joy and solace. On the way back to my room I visit the chapel.

The next day Pastor Wilson visits. In retrospect, it was amazing how he always seemed to show up when I was feeling my lowest, those times when I began thinking I'd had enough already and wanted out of the whole damn mess. How nice of the universe to rearrange itself so that he walked into my room at precisely the moments I need-ed him the most—those times I lay there quietly with tears streaming down my face.

Another video is on the screen now, and one shot dur-ing the previews is that of an alien Spiderman, his bald head marked with dark spiderweb lines. I stare at him in horror and erupt in tears. God, I think, that is what I'm going to look like after the plastic surgery. No, I'll be worse than that; I'll be grotesque in the middle of a living hell. Doug comforts me as usual. That night I watch Nature's

Symphony, a nature scene video set to classical music, and for an hour I'm in heaven.

The next day is the day before surgery. Again, the universe sends out an SOS and all manner of friends and relatives and bosses call to say hello, wish me good luck tomorrow, giving me some of their strength, their energy. During a dressing change, Doug takes a picture of my ugly, putrefying skull for a "before" photo. Later I sit outside again on the patio, gathering strength from nature and everyone passing by. I absorb their energy as they pass; I know I'm going to need it in the weeks ahead. Doug visits again later and doesn't want to leave me at the end of visiting hours. Tomorrow is the big day.

Finally, the waiting game is over.

Doug arrives at 7:00 a.m. the next morning, and at 8:00 a.m. I'm taken to the operating room. What little confidence I have is shot when the anesthesiologist has trouble inserting the breathing tube. First I have to gargle with a thick, foul-tasting antiseptic which makes me start to vomit and gag. Next they spray my throat, then insert a needle to freeze the area. It becomes a nightmare for me; the action turns into slow motion. Suddenly I sit bolt upright on the operating table, gagging, choking, heaving, and crying as operating room staff swarm around me in numbers. Soon the drugs start taking effect. Struggling subsides as I quickly become sedated, falling asleep. They insert the breathing tube, but do it with much difficulty.

In surgery, the neurosurgeon simply lifts the area of rotten, dead skin off the side of my head, revealing the white, synthetic bone patch underneath, which he also removes easily. They debride the area, removing all dead and infected skin and skull bone, and in so doing effectively make the hole in my head larger. Next, the plastic surgeon cuts and rotates scalp (all layers of skin) from the top of my head to the side, to cover the bone hole and brain; then, skin is taken from my right thigh and grafted to the top of the skull to cover the "scalped" area there.

No food. Lots of morphine.

My new headgear is a bandage the size of Marge Simpson's hairdo. I also have a brain drain—a drainage tube complete with large suction ball—inserted into the side of my head to collect excess fluids draining from inside my skull. I look really, really weird. I amuse myself by thinking about accidentally squeezing the suction ball in my hand and sucking my brains out. Wouldn't *that* surprise the doctors?

The next day I am full of aches and pains; my neck is stiff and my right ear is plugged. Morphine is given for the pain. My right thigh is burning. Visible through the transparent bandage, the skin graft donor-site on my thigh looks like a raw steak at the meat counter, red and oozing blood. Neat, in a gory sort of way. Neat meat.

The morphine continues for days, but I don't mind at all. Doug visits, taking me on laps around the hospital floor to keep up my muscle tone. I walk proudly, although slowly and unsteadily, my blood-spotted headdress and all—again a survivor. I'm top heavy, but not in the way I dreamt about.

Later the neurosurgeon visits to tell me a third of my skull will always be bald; the top and back third, to be exact. In my health journal I write, "Dr. S. says BALD!" Now, I'm *really* glad to be on morphine.

Soon a doctor arrives to remove the Jackson Pratt Y Tube brain drain. Doug watches the procedure as the doctor

yanks, tugs, and pulls and pulls a very long, seemingly endless piece of tubing out of my skull. That's something you
don't see every day.

"It hurt to watch," he confesses to me.

"Hurts me more!" I write in my journal. Later in the
day, I'm still seeping drainage behind the ear on the right
side and that scares me.

While attempting to move around the room later the
same day, the gauze covering the transparent bandage
on my donor thigh slips off. The blood seeps out from
under the transparent bandage and flows in rivulets
down my leg. Scared again, I grab some gauze and ring
for the nurse.

My hand is swelling and burning, sore from the IV that
has been in for fourteen days. My thigh donor site is burning. My head hurts. Morphine and antibiotics continue.
Four days post-surgery I am taken off morphine and put
on Demerol for the pain. My journal reads, "Head hurts,
more blood seepage. Feels tight, tingly. Thigh still burning.
Bad bowel cramps. Very tired, sad, depressed. Doug
brings beautiful bouquet from home. So uncomfortable.
No way to lie well. Plastic surgeon was supposed to come
to remove skin dressing, but didn't. Head feels tight and
pulling in dressing. Sore. Pain."

The next day I write, "Frustration. Where is plastics
man? Head pain. Pastor visits again. Bleeding continues.
Start to bleed a lot at side of head. Also, the IV is leaking.
Bleeding continues—more. 9:30: Demerol, Gravol. 1:30
a.m.: Demerol, Gravol. Tired. Need to sleep. Weary."

The day after that, Plastics remove the surgical dressing and take a look. They tell me there's a large bald area

at the top and back of my head, but the graft looks good. I sit stunned, as the reality of the situation finally descends upon me. There's bleeding from the back of my head, but nothing from the side at this point. I've got no appetite. The pastor arrives to discuss my new life, new self-image (being permanently bald, etc.); he's followed by Nurse Robin who's helpful and calming.

Later in the day two neurosurgeons arrive at dressing change time so that they, too, can see my skull. As the bandages are removed, they gaze in shocked silence at my head—stapled, stitched, black and blue, bloody, scabbed, white, wretched. From the look on their faces, I know I am grotesque. The bald spot is at my crown—the best cosmetically, they say. "All I want to do is stop bleeding and heal!" I write.

The following morning I awake dripping blood from the right side of the dressing. Terribly frightening. The dressing is removed and now the back of my head starts to bleed. At 10:00 a.m. I break down. I write, "Cry, sob. Sick of all this blood, blood—three months of it. Nurse consoles. Help me please get well, I plead through wet eyes lifted heavenward. Bad morning, but after drugs, a couple sleeps, and Doug's company I feel better. Cuddle with Doug a bit. Very nice. Miss that a lot."

The next morning there is no blood on the dressing— a very good sign. The neurosurgeons visit. The pastor visits. The volunteer "talker" visits. My psychologist, or "shrink" as I call her, visits. Doug visits. My head injury outreach worker visits. Plastic surgeons visit. Lots of support today. Lots of love going my way. I need it.

As my skin grafts and scalp rotation stabilize and

start healing, attention turns to getting my blood thinness level slowly back up to normal, for the safety of my heart valves. Too fast thinning can cause a lot of bleeding complications on my scalp and internally. They know about excess bleeding from my last surgery and are careful not to repeat it. Lots of visitors again today. Friends, pastor, doctors, Doug. All visitors who see my head today say, "Nice Plastics work," and "Looks better now than before surgery" (when my skin was dead, infected, and putrefying). I take this as a strange compliment. Staples come out today—two really hurt and I cry. Tomorrow the sutures come out.

The following days I play a waiting game—waiting to be released. They want to be sure my blood is thinned to 2.0 before they release me. I write, "Sit and look out windows. Sad but trying to be (crude drawing of happy face) happy. Head aches, burns, crawls, stabs, etc." Head also feels all creepy, crawly, painy, hot, cold, all sensations. I am granted an outing privilege, so Doug and I take advantage of it to have a lovely Greek supper and a walk around the waterfront park. Very romantic. Great to be out. My ensemble is complete with a very large, white gauze turban.

Twenty-three days after being admitted, I'm released. I cry when home comes into view; a walk about the grounds is the first order of the day. I rest, eat, then later go to bed. I write, "Doug makes a big pillowy bed for me. Hard to get comfy as usual, though. Bean-pickers noisy tonight."

It's good to be home.

∾

Things would seem to be picking up now that I'm home, but still there are problems. I write, "Leak! Cry/depressed. Sit stunned, comatose."

And, "Head feels creepy, crawly, painy, hot, cold, all sensations."

Back at the hospital for a follow-up, the Plastics man does a very painful removal of the original dressing tape. "Donor leg site healing well, also crown graft looks good, hair growing; problem with left sutures—infection starting!" I go on a daily regime of 4400 mg. of combined cloxicillan and penicillin V to kill bacteria. I'm told the other antibiotics I was taking were to prevent colonization. (I misinterpret this to mean they would not kill the infection.) All the while my scalp was rotting and pus was flowing, I wasn't on drugs to kill the infection? I assume there was a medical reason for this, but regardless, I do not understand it and it is just too much bad news for me to handle.

Later that day, while at the local blood lab getting my INR checked (blood clotting level for my mechanical heart valves), lab technician Gwen poses an innocent question, "Well, how's your summer going?"

Stunned, I stare at her as my mind does an instant replay of the agony of the last few months. I try to maintain composure, but I can't. I erupt in a major breakdown, run blinded by tears through the waiting room, and stand crying in the hallway just outside the lab doors, reduced to a shuddering, broken soul. "Cry! Breakdown! Infection! Pain!" I write that night in my journal.

And so began the next few months which revolved around playing hide and seek with infection; a few months of constant stress. My journal is ripe with expletives:

"Head weird, itchy, crawly, sore. Thigh donor site ultra-sensitive. Sick of all this!"

"Feel weak, nauseated; wretch from pills."

"Didn't cry today!"

"Head no longer has moonscape quality!"

"Last night, can't get to sleep. Too many flying bugs in room. Doug helps kill them, then I kill the rest as I freak out—sobbing, scared. Doug wakes again and comforts me. I'm nuts!"

"I'm not ready to look—saw glimpse in mirror. Scary!"

"Seepage. Nurse says 'yellow;' I see green—infection. God, I hope not. Pray!"

"Enough! Heal! Please. Pray to God for help. Very depressed, scared. HELP ME!"

"Have good cry in yard. Pray for help!"

"Get sad and cry when looking at models in the Victoria Secret catalogue—none are bald!"

∽

On the morning of September 5th, more than four months after I checked into the hospital April 28th to have my bone flap replaced, I return to the hospital for a final checkup. The plastic surgeon inspects and cleans my head area. I write in my health journal, "Dr. D. removes top scabs—healed underneath; cleans and debrides side wound—only one small suture hole open; applies silver nitrate. Wash head daily, rubbing side with baby shampoo; mineral oil to soften, night before if necessary. Peroxide only when needed. Keep creaming the top (of my head); massage into scalp. No infection evident. Pleased. Some hair loss—nerves will regenerate.

Seepage in three areas will continue. Top will take long to heal."

In the afternoon I visit the neurosurgeon at the hospital. That night I write, "Dr. S. pleased; closes file on me. Have a life before I consider more elective surgery, he says. (Again I think to myself, "Having a bone replaced in the side of your skull is elective?") Can be done in future." And with that, my file was formally closed.

Of course, the irony of this whole experience is that I was better off over four months ago on April 27th, the day *before* I checked into the hospital for the cranioplasty—an operation in which the failure rate odds were one in ten. Obviously, the odds weren't in my favour; I was that one in ten. I had a hole in my head then too, but at least I had a healthy scalp and a full head of hair. Now I'm disfigured, scalped bald, and I'm experiencing increased hair loss on the top right temple area, with hair loss spreading along the scar line to join up with the bald patch. I'd undergone four months of physical and emotional suffering for nothing.

Sometimes, I guess, these things happen.

On November 22nd, I was coughing and blowing my nose because of a cold. "I look down and head is bleeding at side," I write in my journal that night.

On December 25th, Christmas Day 1996, I write, "Get outside midday and early evening. Magical! Full moon tonight. Feel OK. God bless us, everyone."

The View

❧ Nurses

Danielle, Monica, Michelle, Nicole, Lucy, Liza, Shelly, Kelly, Jane, Janet, Greg, Connie, Lisa, Rena, Uli, Tracey, Suzanne, Phyllis, Bea, Lou, Bonnie, Kathy, Beth, Pat, Tracey, Andre, Jake, Shirley…

Registered nurses, student nurses, practical nurses, nurses' aides, nurses' teacher…

Night shift, day shift, afternoon shift.

They come in all shapes and sizes, all manner of attire, and with all personalities. The most important thing you need to know is how to summon them as they whiz by your door on their way to another patient.

You've rung your bell, the nursing station has responded over the speaker (usually in a garbled nearly incomprehensible manner), you've stated your request, and the intercom shuts off. You sit and wait.

And wait. And wait.

Eventually, a harried nurse appears and just as you begin to utter, "Can you please lower the head of my bed?" you get a sinking feeling that perhaps you could have lain there just a little longer, until the nurse made her next *scheduled* stop at your bedside.

The poor creatures, they are all run off their feet, and they will still do the darndest things for you.

It's very important to remember your current nurse's name. I say "current nurse," as in these days of strong nurses' unions and stretched hospital budgets, you will see a veritable symphony of nurses, perhaps three or four today, and rarely the same ones tomorrow.

You must remember their names, so you can summon

them by circumventing the normal buzzer/nurses' station/dispatcher/intercom route, by simply sitting up in bed and, with a steady and purposeful gaze, staring at the doorway. When you see your nurse come into view on her way down the hallway and heading past your door, yell her name at the top of your lungs. "Jane!"

This usually stops her dead in her tracks. Stunned, she looks around to see who called. Repeat her name loudly again, and she will usually come to your bedside. Of course, this method only works if, (1) she hears your voice, and (2) you yell the right name.

You have to be quick and alert to use this method. For many patients this is not an option. Lying in bed moaning, "Nurse... nurse..." does not often bring one. In this case, it is very helpful to have a somewhat mobile and attentive roommate so they can summon help for you.

The proper placement of the help buzzer is very important. I usually had mine tied to the side rail at approximately mid-upper arm position for easiest locating and grabbing, yet still out of the way.

If you have a special request, please remind the nurses of it. Sometimes, with all the best intentions, your nurse will inadvertently forget your special request—perhaps a bed shampoo or another blanket—while on her way to another patient or dealing with a real emergency, such as a patient slip-and-fall or equipment failure alarm. A reminder to your nurse at shift change and when the next new nurse reports to you is your best policy. Don't be afraid to speak up for what you need, and don't be afraid to remind them. Their job is to help you to heal both physically and emotionally.

As many nurses as there were, a few nurses and a few situations stand out in my mind.

It was the first month after the accident, and I hadn't yet had a proper bath. During conversation, when the nurse mentioned she was required to shave men, I piped up that it would be wonderful if she would shave my legs.

With supplies assembled, and me bedded and in position, she began. The first two passes along my left calf went well. Then she got to my shin. Slowly, and with seeming malpurpose, her razor scraped down the top of my shin. "Stop!" I shouted. "You're not skinning a beaver you know!" Surprised at my outburst, she looked down at her handiwork just as red liquid began seeping out of the pores. "It's only blood," she explained defensively and rather annoyed. Rather annoyed, I agreed, but it was after all *my* blood.

In another episode, it had been two weeks since the accident, and I had only been fully conscious for a day or so, when it occurred to me that my hair had never been washed. Being rigged up to monitoring tubes, wires, and IV, the logistics of it eluded me, until a helpful nurse asked me if I would care for a bed shampoo.

I had never heard about anything like that before, but as a former working woman who was used to a shampoo every one or two days, I was desperate to give it a try.

It was 3:00 a.m. when the nurse could spare the time to accommodate me, but since days and nights were a hazy blend at that point, it really didn't matter. I was going nowhere the next morning anyway, so it was agreed.

It took a little hunting and organizing, but she soon appeared with a funny looking, plastic, u-shaped pan, towels, and a pail. Water and shampoo appeared from somewhere and she began.

I lay back in bed into sheer luxury. There is nothing more soothing after the rigors of surgery and guaranteed to help one's recovery than warm water on your body. In this case, it was warm water on my head. The trickling sound, the warmth, the massage, the smell of herbal shampoo—all were heavenly.

Soon it was time to rinse. And rinse she did, over and over again. Six times to be exact. Six pailfuls of reddish-brown water (there was so much dried blood and dirt in my hair from the accident and surgery) until the water rinsed clear. What a treat it was to finally have clean hair. And how grateful I was for the extra time and tender loving care the nurse lavished on me.

Nurses are a patient's maid, servant, friend, medical advisor, teacher, helpmate, mother, psychologist, and comic relief. They will do practically anything for you. But as in any profession, there is sometimes a bad apple, and sometimes just a bad circumstance. In my case, the two combined to create a personal tragedy for me.

It was a week following my cranioplasty surgery, in May '96, to fill the hole left in my skull resulting from the December '94 accident. All week long I'd had numerous nurses having to soak the gauze dressing off my scabbed head in order to do a dressing change. The sutures and staple sites were still seeping blood, and that blood was drying into the gauze, making the dressing extremely stuck to my skull.

An evening nurse was doing the dressing change prior to my bedtime. She acted a bit clumsy, rough, and hurried, like the proverbial bull in a china shop, I thought. Sloppily she dropped the scissors, then knocked some dressings off the table onto the floor. Tensing up, I cautioned her, "You have to soak the dressing off my head as it gets stuck." She peeked under the dressing a couple times, said, "It's OK," then... rip! She yanked it off.

"Oh, it's starting to bleed!" she exclaimed, and with that put her palm onto my tender, surgical head and pressed to stop the bleeding. She pressed and pressed and pressed. It felt as if the fresh staples were being pushed clear through my skull. The pain was excruciating.

"Stop!" I screamed.

"I have to stop the bleeding," she snapped.

"Stop, you're hurting me!" I wailed.

She wrapped my head into a gauze turban, a very, very tight one, but soon it was soaked with blood.

She removed it and rewrapped, this time a little looser. Nevertheless, my head was still throbbing from the onslaught. When she left, I called my husband, sobbing uncontrollably, hysterical about the pain. "She hurt me... so... bad..." my voice trailed off as I cried.

This episode was really unfortunate for me, for at that point I lost almost all faith in the medical profession. I trusted no one from then on who was a doctor, a surgeon, or a nurse. I became hyper-vigilant, and every action of any consequence or possible consequence was suspect, questioned, feared. I had gone to a very bad, very lonely place for a patient to be.

After talking with Doug, I paged the nurses' desk to ask for painkillers, but I didn't want Nurse Connie to bring them. I didn't want her to touch me ever again, I told them. Unbelievably, Nurse Connie arrived with a needle. I cried, "I don't want you to touch me! You hurt me."

She replied, "I didn't do it on purpose, you know."

To make a long story short, my family and I forbade her to come into my room again, and when I returned two months later to have the damage repaired by more surgery, she was banned from entering my room.

The event resulting in the actual damage to my head—a large haematoma that eventually led to serious infection, bone patch deterioration, and the death of parts of my scalp—became known as "the incident" in the ward.

When I think about Connie's full head of wavy red hair, in contrast with my resulting skin grafts and scalp rotation, and the huge, permanent bald spot, I feel a little angry. But Connie was the rare exception. The other nurses were gentle and caring. Many times I was comforted, and many times we laughed.

What it comes down to is this—your nurse is your lifeline. She is the link to all hospital services. She will do almost anything for you, if you ask and if she has the time. Handle her with kid gloves and thank her often. Realize she is only human and is just trying to do her job.

Nurses are a marvelous group of people. But don't take my word for it. Nurses scored highest when Canadians were polled in April 2000 on which professions they placed their trust in. Rightly so.

❧ Jargon

After you are hit and run over by a van, the interesting phrase "road pizza" is useful in describing your predicament. This is a much better phrase than the popular "road kill," which in my case was incorrect, thank goodness. Besides, "road pizza" is much more colourful.

The phrase "road pizza" was created (in the hospital by Doug, once I was awake and communicating) to quickly describe the condition of lying on the street with tire marks down myself, with my innards oozing outwards. It provided the right amount of levity at the time, and made it easier to refer to my fresh, post-accident condition in a lighter way. While the phrase sounds a bit harsh, it worked for me. It was our own brand of soft-speak jargon.

The same tactic is used by the medical profession as a way of clouding the issue, softening the truth, calling a spade a stick with a rounded thing on the end. This is by no means an attack or a complaint towards the medical establishment; it is merely my observation.

Here are some instances of bonafide, soft-speak jargon that were used by doctors and nurses.

After the surgery, for instance, the doctors reported to my husband that they had to "paralyze" me. What this meant was, that in order to keep me absolutely still for a long period of time they medically induced a paralysis—an unconsciousness—no movement whatsoever. They had used an accurate concise term to describe a complicated condition.

Later on, when the orthopedic surgeon made his rounds, during his verbal inspection of me he uttered the term "exit site." This is a most descriptive and efficient terminology to describe the wound location where a broken bone had protruded through the skin. My two "exit sites" referred to two scars where: (1) my broken thigh bone stuck out of my skin; and (2) my broken elbow bone stuck out of my skin. To me, "exit site" sounded comical, as if my bones could decide to leave or try to escape on their own through a special neon-lit doorway. I thought this phrase to be soft-speak jargon at its finest.

During my hospital recuperation, another soft-speak jargon emerged. I was given a pill daily that was termed a "muscle relaxant." It was usually given at bedtime and seemed to put me to sleep. This drug was once also administered when a severe bout of anxiety during a cognitive rehabilitation session raised my heart rate too high. It quickly reduced the heavy, quick pounding and relaxed me. Yes, it was a muscle relaxant, but something was bugging me, so I asked, "Is this a tranquilizer?"

"It's a muscle relaxant," they responded.

Post-hospital, while talking with a pharmacist, she referred to the drug as a potentially addictive tranquilizer, which is the same thing really. But "muscle relaxant" sounds good—"tranquilizer" sounds bad; so the patients heard the soft-speak jargon version. Over the next three weeks I weaned myself off the drug and, admittedly, at times it was difficult to cut back. I had become just a bit addicted, but definitely for medicinal purposes. I had the prescriptions to prove it.

Jargon, especially the soft-speak brand, is necessary in the life-and-death hospital environment where the truth is often painful, where the truth is not worth worrying about, or when the truth is just too time-consuming.

You need a lot of coping strategies when you spend long periods of time in the hospital. Humorous jargon, like "road pizza," is a godsend, even if you do have to make it up yourself. It was one coping strategy that worked for me.

❧ Spouse and Caregiver

I was blessed. When God handed out loving mates, he gave me Doug.

If there was any one reason why I survived not only open-heart surgery in August '92, but this near-fatal accident of December '94, other than my own sheer will to live and incredible surgeons, it was Doug. As devastated as he was by my accident, he somewhere found the strength to take control. He was, and still is over two years later, my main caregiver.

What did he do? Let me tell you:

1. He visited me every day I was in the hospital. This was no easy task. It meant a drive to Kingston and back, a 215 km round trip every day, through all kinds of weather, and despite trying to hold down a job. (He later lost that job because of too much time off.) The first week I really wasn't aware of him being there—but after that, he became my knight in shining armour. I eagerly awaited his visits.

2. Because of the bright hospital lights, the strange sounds, and my discomfort and inactivity, I was having trouble sleeping through the nights during the first month. What did Doug do? He brought my favourite nighttime sleeping potion—hot milk and Ovaltine prepared fresh in the nurses' microwave. That did the trick.

3. Because my arm was in a splint, I had trouble maneuvering the dinner fork to my mouth. To remedy this, Doug brought me a bright purple, deep-bowled airplane-shaped spoon. It not only made eating more fun, but food didn't spill out of it onto my lap, or worse, inside my neck brace.

4. My appetite was poor, so I had little interest in the hospital food and my spirits were down. To remedy that, Doug appeared one day with a lovely ice cream sundae— just what the doctor forgot to order. Another day Doug presented me with an instant-win bingo card and a pizza. Now, that was a party.

5. What else did he do? Very often at night he'd call at bedtime, just to say goodnight and that he loved me. I adored that.

6. Life gets very boring, very quickly once your condition improves to the point that you're awake and out of pain for the most part. Being unable to walk and get around caused me a lot of frustration. To fix that, Doug bundled me into the wheelchair and gave me the royal tour. Around the hospital corridors we went, up and down the elevators, exploring other floors, the cafeterias, the gift shops, and so on. The breeze on my face felt great, and because Doug always liked driving fast it was quite exciting at times. When we'd return to the room, I felt refreshed from the ride.

7. Being bedridden, a back rub felt wonderful. Doug excelled at that, having strong muscular hands. Heaven.

8. Early on, during my weaker times, the feel of Doug's warm hand on mine and the soothing stroking of

my head helped to calm and reassure me. "Very soothing," I'd whisper time and time again.

9. Backgammon was a game we enjoyed many years ago, and it was just perfect for the hospital situation. Hoping to take advantage of my weakened state, his high dreams of victory were dashed when I continued to win. Although very tiring, it was fun and helped to pass some time.

10. One thing a patient needs is a lot of hugs and a lot of laughter. Doug supplied both of these. Each visit, he'd eagerly await to hear my commentary on the day. I found the best strategy was to look for the funny side to everything that happened. With hand movements, facial expressions, and embellishments, my stories entertained him and his laughter was infectious. He always saw the funny side of things and kept me laughing, too. His news of life back at home kept me up-to-date and helped minimize the feelings of isolation.

11. He paced me. He'd monitor my visitors, and would tactfully ask them to end their visit when he noticed I was becoming tired. And back at home, he'd remind me when to lie down, rest, or do something else. He knew that if I became overtired I would get either sad, weepy, or angry; or else, the next day I'd have no energy at all and would be sad, weepy, or angry about that. If you're thinking I got sad, weepy, and angry a lot—you're right. But Doug's monitoring helped control it.

12. My passions are: (1) nature, (2) my home, (3) gardening, (4) my dogs/walking—not necessarily in that order. The first year, however, due to my orthopedic and

head injuries, bending down or over to garden was a problem. What did Doug do? He fashioned some tools to help me. He took a sturdy wooden chair and cut the legs off halfway so I could sit close to the earth. He also took two garden hand-tools and inserted long wooden poles (old broom handles) to lengthen them, making it easier for me to reach. What superb joy it was to feel the sun on my face and smell the soil as I did a little bit of gardening.

13. He pestered me. It is two years post-accident, and my brain injury deficits have been assessed and documented. Almost from the start they were evident. The classics: short-term memory loss, mental and physical fatigue, sensory overload, difficulty concentrating and initiating, etc. Right from the start, Doug hammered into me day after day, "write it down," or "make a list," or "do a schedule." At first, I thought that since I wasn't working, I didn't have anything important enough to schedule or write down. It seemed rather elementary. But I was in denial. It soon became apparent my brain was failing me; the simplest tasks of getting through the day and doing not a lot of anything did take some planning. Thanks to Doug's urgings and to the Head Injury Outreach Worker, I acquired a day planner and was instructed on its use. I began to schedule, keep track of my many doctor appointments and meetings, make "to-do" lists and just generally write things down. Things like "laundry," "water plants," "mail letters," "pay bills," "call friend," "take form to doctor for signing" are written down and checked off when completed, giving me a sort of structure to my day and a sense of purpose and accomplishment. Now, every evening Doug asks what I have on for the next day, or if

I'm still in bed when he leaves in the morning, he just glances at the day planner for an update.

14. He hugged me—a lot. Lots of times I'd burst into tears for no apparent reason. The professionals call it labile emotions, resulting from the brain injury. Usually it was some sound or image that triggered a subconscious fear, sense of loss, or horror within me. Sometimes it would be in frustration or anger at not being able to do something I'd previously been able to. He'd look at me and ask, "What? What is it?" in a calm, reassuring voice, then come over and hug me while I'd blabber out something or other between sobs. "It's OK," he'd say. "It's only a movie," or offer some sort of down-to-earth remedy such as, "Just ask for help. I'll help you." After some hugging and gentle stroking, my crying would be over; I'd be calmer and more secure in his love.

And perhaps this last point, #14, is the one that helped me the most—his acceptance of my weakest moments when my fears and losses would flood to the surface and dissolve into tears.

Those hugs—they were, and still are—the best help.

❧ The Closed Door

I remember the regular fire drills we had at school when I was young; we'd all stand obediently and walk outside in an orderly manner, hang around the schoolyard for a while, then head back inside to our respective classes.

In the hospital, it doesn't quite happen like that.

First, you hear the alarm start ringing. Then, you look at your roommate in the next bed, begin speculating what the noise is all about, and look towards the doorway. Next you hear increased activity in the hallway, and a methodical slamming as hospital staff make their way down the corridor closing each door, one by one as they pass.

"I wonder why they closed our door?" you think. Then the thought occurs to you, "It must be a fire!" Or a fire drill, you hope. You pray it's not a fire for the simple reason that the logistics of escaping escapes you. "How will they save me?" crosses your mind. "I can't walk, I'm strapped in the bed, and I'm attached to a machine and an IV. I'm quite helpless."

You hear the fire engine sirens getting louder and louder as they race towards the hospital. "It *is* a fire!" you exclaim to your roommate. You look at each other with eyes now as big as saucers. You wait and listen. After what seems like a long time, the din in the hallway subsides and, one by one, the reopening of doors can be heard throughout the ward. "Smoke in the kitchen. No fire," is the word. Soon, things are back to normal and the predictable monotony of the hospital resumes. However, thanks to that exciting episode, our day at the hospital has been made just a little more interesting, and we have a whole new story to tell our loved ones when they visit or call.

One evening something strange happened. It took me a while to notice it, but I slowly became aware of increased activity in the hallway, followed by the methodical closing of doors. That's weird, I thought. I didn't hear any alarm. Activity level in the hallway increased yet again, and through the little window on my door I could see the heads and shoulders of people passing by. But something was strange; it looked like a parade, not only of doctors or nurses, but all kinds of people in all manner of attire passing by my door. No siren. Closed doors. Lots of people. Soon the activity ended; the reopening of doors began, and things returned to normal.

Later that evening word got around—a patient on the floor had died. I put two and two together. The closed doors allowed the procession of family and friends following the deceased being wheeled down the corridor, a measure of privacy in their grief, while acting as a protective shield to patients, who, unaware, lay quietly healing in their beds behind closed doors. An eerie situation that heightened my awareness of the life-and-death reality that is hospital life.

From then on, closed hospital room doors became a grim omen that I passed with head bowed reverently, just in case.

❧ "If Only I Hadn't" Syndrome

I guess it's part guilt and part an attempt to explain the unexplainable, that leads many people to strangely say, "If only I hadn't... (such and such)... you wouldn't have had the accident."

I call it the "If Only I Hadn't Syndrome." In the first several months following the accident, it ran rampant.

My boss confessed, "If only I hadn't put pressure on everyone to sell, sell, sell Christmas and Boxing Day ads, then you wouldn't have been out there pounding the pavement, and you wouldn't have been hit."

One of my customers confessed, "If only I had been in that morning when you called on me, we would have had our meeting, you would have been delayed, and you wouldn't have had the accident."

Another customer confessed, "If only I'd had the advertising copy ready for you when you arrived, you wouldn't have been delayed, and you wouldn't have been hit."

An ex-colleague confessed, "If only I hadn't bumped into you and stopped to chat that morning just before you crossed the street, you wouldn't have been delayed and you would be OK today."

My mind wanders… "If only I hadn't been thinking about last minute Christmas gifts yet to buy as I crossed the street, perhaps I might have heard the van barreling down on me." (Yes, I did look both ways before stepping off the curb after the little man in the traffic light said "walk," but one doesn't continue looking both ways while crossing the street; at least I've never seen anyone doing this. *Now* I do it.)

In this case, it was probably a blessing in disguise. If I had heard the van, I might have turned, or I might have stiffened in fear, thereby causing more severe injuries. As it was, I was relaxed and oblivious—no doubt the best way to be hit, thrown, and run over by a full-size van.

The infiniteness of this "If only I hadn't syndrome" is quite mind-boggling:

If only I hadn't gone to work that day… if only I hadn't moved to The County… if only I hadn't been born… then this wouldn't have happened to me.

The first several months after the accident, all I could think and say was, "Why me?" The question played over and over in my mind. In fact, many people ask themselves that same question when faced with major upheavals in their lives.

Of course, what we all know (or at least what I know now) is that everything happened that day as it was supposed to happen. There was nothing anyone could have done differently to change the outcome, because that was the only outcome possible. Everything had gone along as planned. Everyone did as they were supposed to do. Tough plan for me, yes, but who said life's plan is easy?

What happened to me, happened for a reason. In retrospect, after a lot of thinking and reading, I can say that.

The process leading up to this realization has been a long one. Accepting that "everything happened that day as it was supposed to" takes a great leap of faith and insight.

A lot of time quietly convalescing at home, thinking and reading was responsible; it was a time when my spiritual beliefs were challenged and developed. The accident was the catalyst.

❧ Shared Experiences

One thing you can be sure of, once you are involved in an accident or are fighting a major illness, you need to speak to others who are going through the same things as you are. We find comfort in this. Although each situation is different, we share common physiological reactions and emotions. It is somehow comforting to know we are not alone in our suffering.

Whether in the hospital, support group, or rehabilitation centre, I discovered there is a strange sort of one-upmanship operating to establish who has suffered the most. Comments like: "I was in the hospital for three months," versus "I was in the hospital for six months;" or "I was hit by a car," versus "I was hit, thrown, and run over by a full-size van;" or "I was unconscious for three days," versus "I was unconscious for three weeks;" or "I broke two ribs," as opposed to "I had an open compound fracture of the right leg and an open compound fracture of the right arm" are common.

Is it to elicit the most pity or to brag about our survival skills that we do this? Either way, they make for great stories. Let's face it, this major illness or accident is probably the most significant event that's happened to you—the most intense, the most exciting, and the most horrific. Things have happened to you that the inexperienced cannot hope to understand. Only fellow survivors who have suffered can fully share what you have been through.

That's one reason support groups exist. They are a means of accessing people of similar medical histories. By informally discussing your problems, fears, and coping strategies a lot of helpful information is shared.

Further into your recovery process, as you heal, you may require less support. Conversely, if your healing process drags on, you may find continued interaction with a support group necessary.

Just talking to friends and acquaintances—your major unofficial support group—can be revealing. For instance, one girlfriend I hadn't spoken to for a while had several ear operations to remedy a constant ringing, but to no avail. Another friend was in a horse and buggy accident on her farm and, while now recovered, still has to sleep with many pillows to help ease her bones. Talking to my friends helped me sympathize with them, turn my attention outward and away from myself for awhile.

But you know, no one really wants to know about the infinite, minute details of your accident more than someone who has had similar problems, similar experiences, or similar losses. And here again, that strange sort of one-upmanship arises, where you keep tally in your mind of who's "the winner"—who has suffered the most.

There is a weird irony in this game, whereby the loser is really the winner. "On a scale of one to ten, I was an eight," I think. "I was a five," the other chap thinks. Ten is dead. He wins. Strange.

Without a doubt, the best place to share your experiences is in the hospital. What a goldmine. Everyone here is sick or hurt, and all the details of your experiences are fresh in your mind because they are happening to you now. The immediacy of it all gives the hospital game of one-upmanship a special intensity.

Not knowing how long your hospital stay will be, there is an urgency to share your story with your roommates, with people lined up at x-ray, with other patients in the TV/lounge room, etc.

And again, you listen to their story. They listen to yours. You make the tally in your mind—I'm a seven, they're only a two. Twos hold less interest for you. You want to speak to another seven, or a six, or an eight. Can't speak to a ten—they're dead. And all the twos are being discharged tomorrow. They're no fun.

∽

I found that two common themes emerged during my sharing of experiences.

One question was, "Why did this happen to me?" That seems like a hard one, but with hindsight and the magic of healing or "moving on," you will observe that your illness is a catalyst to your personal growth—almost like a turning point. One moment you're this person doing this with your life, then, the next, you're a different person doing something completely different.

Those who believe in fate will have no problem with the concept that it's all happened for a reason. If you're a skeptic and you don't believe in fate, it's a lot harder. But even skeptics often become believers in fate, and it usually depends on the severity of their own eventual sickness or injury. Maybe that's because the sicker we are, the more time we have to think while recovering. Then, the natural thought process is to ask, "Why?" Others are simply introspective by nature, and automatically think about these life issues.

Hindsight is probably the best revealer of the theory of fate. During the course of your recovery, take the time to look at what has happened, speculate why, then sit back and observe the many changes that occur in your life. When you change because of your sickness or accident, others around you have to change too. You are the impetus that makes those who interact with you every day, interact with you differently. This resulting change in them is an opportunity for growth—new responsibilities, new emotions, new experiences, and new plans. It's a period of healing for all.

The other overall common theme that revealed itself

was concerning the pain. When I was hit by the van, I felt no pain. Imagine! One patient, a fellow who was deliberately bumped off his motorcycle at high speeds by another vehicle, incurring numerous external and internal injuries, felt no initial accident pain. And another patient, a girl who was crushed and pinned in another motorcycle accident, felt no pain.

When the pain is too horrible, too intense, it is shunted to your deepest recesses, not of your mind, but of your body. Cellular memory they call it. Memories too painful to be recalled by the conscious mind are locked away inside.

Of course, there is the pain of recuperation, recovery, rehabilitation, and of managing your disabilities or injuries. But the pain of the actual moment is blocked out. This "no pain" phenomenon, obviously a latent survival strategy in us all, was the most wondrous discovery of my many shared experiences.

❧ Roommates

What can I say about roommates? If you're in anything other than a private room—you've got one. And with all my hospital stays, I've had some interesting ones.

One roommate was an escape artist. Helen would never stay where the nurses put her, especially when told to stay put. And despite my urgings to stay put, she would get up and wander. She was very weak, fragile, and unsteady on her feet, but able to untie any restraint device the nurses could come up with. Whether freed from her bed or her chair, she would suddenly be up and wandering about, sometimes leaving the room. She would usually make her reappearance shortly thereafter, escorted by a nurse.

Another roommate, Bonnie, arrived at the Rehab ward already equipped with a walker; but walking had nothing to do with it. She used the walker like a giant scooter—one leg perched on the seat while the other propelled her through the hospital halls at top speed. I hadn't noticed at first that the leg perched on the seat was a stump; that's all that was left of her leg after a serious motorcycle accident. She was back to heal an infection and for the fitting of a new prosthetic leg.

I soon came to learn she was a veteran of many hospital stays and had developed a coping strategy. When Bonnie "moved in" she came equipped with all the comforts—extra pillows, potato chips, craft projects, etc.—and made herself at home, curled up in front of her rented TV. I was impressed by her relaxed complacency.

This next roommate needed some TLC. Heather was an elderly woman whose husband had died not too long ago, and she had since lost the will to live. Her busy daughter had little time for her and, from what I could gather, they weren't close.

When I first arrived at the hospital, Heather ate, slept, and spent all her time sitting in the chair with her feet up. She had serious problems with the nerves in the back of her legs, and as a result her legs were painful and swollen. The nurses would arrive at pill time and leave pills for her to take, a total of twenty-six per day. She'd take the pills, eat her meal, then shortly thereafter vomit them up. Sometimes she'd hazard standing up on her own, and some of these times she fell. I'd be busy constantly with the buzzer, summoning the nurses whenever she needed help. At night I'd hear her praying out loud, "Dear God, please take me tonight." This was distressing for me; I cried a lot for Heather.

Then I took a new tactic.

I began telling her that sitting up all day and night in the same chair was the worst thing she could do for her legs. I said she should try to go for a walk to help her legs pump away the excess fluids, and try to lie down flat at night to take the pressure off her hips and thighs. I told her to ask the nurse to write down what pills she was taking and why, and what pills she could begin to cut back. To my delight, she began to do all this—a sign that her will to live was returning. Then, one night she got up the courage to try sleeping in her hospital bed, a veritable miracle, and as I watched her sleeping soundly from across the room, I cried quiet tears of joy. Even better than that, it was the start of her recovery and eventual return home.

∾

Roommates come in all shapes, sizes, and conditions. The important thing to remember is they are probably scared and hurting, much like you.

Right now if you can, turn your head and look over at the person in the bed beside you. Wait until they turn their head to look over at you. Now smile. Chances are your roommate needed that friendly smile and chances are, if they were able to, they smiled back. Now don't you both feel better?

Smile and take interest in your roommate's situation. A little compassion goes a long way.

❧ Fears and Phobias

Getting hit, thrown, and run over by a van does something strange to your brain. That massive trauma created fears and phobias of all sorts in me.

Simple things like the fear of further surgery or getting hurt again are obvious, but I developed some specialized fears leading me to observe that phobias come tailor-made. Ambulance sirens, crossing the street, watching TV, soft spots, being a passenger, and daydreaming all took on heightened meaning.

Ambulance Sirens: After being hit I awoke briefly. Although unable to focus, I sensed a faceless crowd huddled around me, then heard someone say the ambulance had been called. The ambulance arrived quickly they say. I didn't hear the sirens; I was in shock and lay there on the ground. The sirens which announced my journey to Belleville General Hospital, then to Kingston General, and everything they signified, inflicted great damage to my psyche—damage that would often reveal itself during the months ahead.

Shortly after my release from hospital, while riding through town with Doug en route to see the family doctor, an ambulance overtook us, speeding by with sirens wailing. As a severe panic swept over me, I burst into uncontrollable sobs of childlike fear. Doug pulled the car over to the side of the road. "It's OK, it's OK," he comforted, hugging me close to him until my crying stopped. It took over seven months' time for my violent reaction to the sound of sirens to end.

Crossing the Street: I had looked both ways before stepping off the curb and was midway through the crossing. I didn't hear or feel the van come from behind, hitting my right side. But for about six months after, when being escorted across the street, I would freeze whenever I saw a car or truck or bus coming towards me. Sometimes I would be in the middle of the traffic lane and would stand staring at the oncoming vehicle. A tug on my arm from my escort would be all it took to jog me back to reality and lead me to safety.

I got out of that habit eventually, but developed an alternate reaction. In these episodes, I wouldn't look both ways before leaving the curb, but would boldly step out into traffic, much to the shock of my escort. This feeling of invincibility was far more dangerous than my previous freeze reactions, and lasted a few months as well. Now, almost three years later, I look both ways before leaving the curb and continue checking both ways for traffic as I cross. (This constant turning of my head back and forth is difficult because it throws me off balance, balance which is already shaky at best due to brain injury.)

TV Shows: For many reasons, it's unfortunate that modern television is so violent. As disgusting as it is normally, for a person who's undergone severe trauma, the impact of TV violence is sometimes quite overwhelming. Actors getting hit by cars or falling from tall buildings generated fear and horror, causing me to look away, unable to hold back the tears. This fear response lasted several months, but eventually subsided as I became numbed through over-saturation of violence, much like I had been before the accident. (Much like everyone is continually being conditioned to escalating scenes of violence.) What hasn't left me is an oversensitivity to anyone on TV who is experiencing pain or seemingly unending adversity, in which case, compassionate tears flow easily.

Soft Spot: The removal of a piece of skull bone just above my right ear to allow for brain swelling post-accident, has left me with a large "soft spot" much like a baby's, except mine will never grow over. The skin covering it has eventually grown strong, and my hair has finally grown in, but I always sense my extreme vulnerability. It doesn't matter where I go—to a restaurant, store, movie theatre—anywhere there is activity and people around me, I am afraid of getting poked in my soft spot. Fear of falling, or bumping my head into an open cupboard door, or getting poked in the head by a branch swaying in the wind are all real threats to my safety. These cause a sort of super-carefulness, an over-cautiousness, or hyper-vigilance, which reduces the pleasure of everyday activities. Spontaneity and abandon are forbidden, as each setting is assessed for danger before I enter. It is as if my brain is dangerously exposed as a tempting target; and of course it is, which only heightens my sense of fragility.

Car travel: It was a beautiful sunny day, fifteen months after the accident, and we were on our way to enjoy a pancake breakfast at the maple sugar bush. I was gazing out the side window at the scenery flying by, when Doug's arm suddenly slammed across my chest as he braked hard to avoid a stopped car ahead. Mesmerized, I watched the bumper ahead closing in at me, then looked away to await the inevitable disaster. Luckily, Doug's artful braking and steering onto the shoulder got us around the car safely. I sat in shock as we continued in silence. "Do something!" my body silently commanded.

I began slow, measured breathing to calm my heart and my brain, but soon an extreme weak sensation overcame me, sinking me deeply—weakly—into the car seat. I sat quietly, but only for a moment. It surged from deep inside, rising like vomit, breaking out of my throat and past my lips—a sound so forlorn, so beaten, so mournful, I wondered where it came from. I shuddered as a series of hysterical sobs and moans, direct from the soul, racked my small frame. I surrendered to these waves of agony and fear, releasing the horror of that December '94 accident, which every cell in my body remembered so well. Doug sat quietly as my grief slowly subsided. After some time I calmed, and we continued on our way.

Daymares: I coined this phrase myself, a cross between daydreams and nightmares. No doubt they originate from deep-seated fears, combined with my near-death experience, and an active imagination. The best way to describe them would be to give you a comparable scenario. Let's pretend I'm walking my dog down the road. As a car approaches, I gaze at it and my mind starts to wander. Suddenly I see a horrific accident in my mind's eye. I see the car speeding towards me, hitting my dog, and pulling me along with it as I hold onto its leash. I end up wrapped around a tree and see my arm, torn off, but still attached to the leash, hanging in the nearby bush.

This sounds horrible, and it is. The daymare lasts less than a minute. I pull myself back to reality and shake my head while saying out loud, "No, that's not going to happen."

Daymares can occur a few times a day, or I can go for a few days without one. The situation is always somehow related to what I am doing at the moment, and always ends in my death or near death and physical mangling.

Lately, I have taken a new tactic that seems to be working. When I feel a daymare coming on and, if I can remember in time, I say to myself something like, "I don't want these daymares anymore. They're not helpful to me and they're not healthy. So please stay away." I've noticed I'm having less of them now. When I do have one I repeat, "No, that's not going to happen. I'm going to be all right."

I hope so.

❧

All those gruesome daymares were upsetting for me; if you're experiencing similar problems, I'm sure they're distressing for you, too. From my experience, it seems you just have to wait it out. It takes a lot of time for the horror to work itself naturally out of your system, and that may include psychotic episodes like I experienced: screaming, crying spells, curling up in the fetal position, nightmares, etc. In the meantime, you may need help developing coping strategies or just talking it over with someone, perhaps a clinical psychologist or rehabilitation therapist. Tell your doctor what you're dealing with; he'll be able to refer you to somebody. There are a lot of people to call on who can help, so please don't be afraid to ask.

✺ The Brick Wall—Exhaustion

Sudden, total exhaustion—the brick wall, the therapist called it. When energy output outstrips energy reserves. She scribbled four letters on a piece of paper and held it in front of my face. WHOA! she'd written. Slow down, stop, rest.

You've heard this one before: "Rest in bed. Keep warm." Good advice on how to deal with the common cold, but what does it have to do with healing or with the brick wall mentioned above? It has a lot to do with energy. Laying still, no exertion, and conserving heat all preserve bodily energy, allowing the body to channel all its energy into getting well. The brick wall is merely the screeching halt induced by exhaustion. Sorry, no more energy. Out of gas. Simple as that.

One thing I learned well is that healing requires tremendous amounts of energy. For the first six months following the accident, my body was busy rebuilding bone cells, muscle cells, blood cells, and nerve cells. Using more energy for healing than my body was generating, I dropped from 108 pre-accident pounds to a mere 89 pounds.

To stabilize my energy drain and try to reverse it, I started taking a liquid nutritional supplement (similar to Boost or Ensure) to increase my calorie intake. (A calorie is a unit measurement of heat, or energy.) I continued with this supplementation for about three months, until my weight hit 100. It is now almost two years later and my weight is 110 pounds. Finally, people tell me I look healthy.

Imagine, one day you're walking 4 kilometres a day in high heels, selling newspaper advertising to downtown retailers before going home and walking your dogs for another mile; then, three months later (in my case, after the accident) you exhaust yourself getting to the kitchen table to eat, so you have to lay down and rest. The brick wall—you just hit it. And what if six months later you take an escorted walk across the yard and back; exhausted, you have to lie down. Wham, you hit the brick wall again. And what if one-and-a-half years later, after you wake up, get washed, dressed, and have breakfast, you have to lie down because, bang, you've hit the wall one more time.

That brick wall did terrible things to my mind. Layers upon layers of tearful frustration resulted from not being able to do what I wanted, when I wanted, and for as long as I wanted. I could only do them when and for as long as my body allowed.

Today, I'm careful to stop short of the brick wall; the day's activities are planned, allowing for two rest breaks daily. I've learned that two major activities a day are the maximum for me. If I do three, such as physio at home in the morning, a trip to town in the afternoon, and a meeting or social visit in the evening—it is too much. No time for two rests, and the next day I'm too tired to do anything.

Respecting the brick wall helps me live a better life. It will help you, too.

❧ The Injuries

It's two-and-a-half years after the accident, and Doug and I are in a movie theatre watching one of those now-so-common disaster films. The hero, get this, is being crushed in a truck, trapped inside a collapsing mine shaft within a mountain that's in volcanic eruption. The camera shot rests on his arm and focuses in on a piece of clean white bone sticking out through a bloody sleeve. Of all the disastrous moments we've witnessed so far in this film, that's the scene which affects everyone. "Eeeeewwwww," the audience gasps, turning their heads in horror so as to avert their eyes from the image of the protruding bone.

I look at Doug and whisper, "Open compound fracture. Been there. Done that."

"Exit site," says Doug, pointing at the split and bleeding skin on the screen.

We look at each other and laugh.

It's good we can laugh about it now, but on that winter day in late '94, no one was laughing.

Minutes after the accident, the ambulance rushed to Belleville General Hospital, delivering me to the Emergency Room. My coat was removed, and blood-soaked clothes cut away. The ER doctor assessed my condition, and when the x-ray technician asked what to x-ray, the orders were, "Everything."

On return to the ER, cuts (called lacerations) and scrapes (called abrasions) were treated, and bandages applied to stop the bleeding of my broken elbow and leg. My mouth and cheeks were swollen and all my teeth were loose. I was a mess.

During all this, I remarkably managed to moan, "Tell the doctors I'm on blood thinners," and repeatedly complained of a rushing sound inside my head, behind my right ear. Taking heed, the doctors sent me back to x-ray for a head scan.

The brain injury was obvious. Unequipped to deal with an intracerebral bleed, the doctor looked at Doug, said, "We can't handle this," and ordered me sent to Kingston General for emergency surgery.

(They tell me I was a little out of control. I was probably hysterical, in a non-conscious sort of way, but I don't remember any of it. Being oblivious to what goes on around you at times like this is a godsend.)

You may be wondering what happens to a body when it's been in such an accident. My injuries were:

- Open compound fracture, right femur (mid shaft);
- Open compound fracture, right elbow;
- Basal skull fracture;
- Intracerebral bleed, right temporal lobe (intra-parenchymal bleed);
- Underwent right craniotomy for evacuation of the hemorrhage;
- Massive tongue and pharyngeal hematoma;
- Numerous lacerations.

That's what the hospital reports read. I've listed the direct, at time of impact injuries, but there's also the matter of what I call indirect injuries—those conditions that manifest at a later date, but result from the original accident. In my case, it was the disastrous end-result of an operation, one-and-a-half years post-accident, to repair the hole in my skull where a 4 inch piece of bone had been removed to allow for brain swelling.

During that operation, synthetic bone was molded to fit the hole in my skull and glued into place. Unfortunately, over the next week, infection set in, infecting the bone patch and killing all the skin covering it. This new problem was corrected by another surgery two months later to: remove the synthetic bone; remove the rotted skin; rotate the scalp to shift good healthy scalp from the top of my head to the side of my head; and take a skin graft from my right thigh to cover the now exposed bone on the top of my head.

This whole procedure left me worse off. With a concave soft spot, I was still without skull bone on the right side of my head, but now I also had a large, permanently bald patch on the top and back third of my head.

In time the broken elbow healed, although it is not as strong as before. The broken leg healed with the aid of a steel rod and pins still intact at its core, with recurring pain at the knee and hip. The skull and scalp healed, but with the scarring and malformation stunningly observable.

But, there's more. There's the other damage the accident caused—the residual emotional, cognitive, physical, and functional damage.

I made a list one tearful day, almost two years after my accident. On it I wrote what damage the accident caused. This is what I wrote:

Physical Problems:

- pain-sensations in scalp (top and right side);
- face bones ache in bad weather (right side, cheek);
- tingly/numb right facial area (triangular), lip to eye;
- wrinkled retina, right eye (sees horizontal and vertical lines wavy);

- degree of colour-blindness (right eye);
- right eye sees images 20 percent larger, as well as wavy distortions;
- wear glasses always now to compensate for bad right vision;
- field of vision reduced in upper left quadrant in both eyes;
- elbow aches with excess use, weight; weather affects it;
- knee/hip aches with excess use, and bad weather;
- reduced agility, flexibility, mobility, balance;
- numerous scars, lacerations;
- permanent scalp and skull disfigurement;
- crooked jaw/smile, loss of facial symmetry;
- no mobility in upper right side of face, and right eyebrow is static; cannot move right eyebrow and forehead;
- surgeries pending, three to correct resulting conditions;
- dizziness/balance—feelings of being off-balance; fast head movements, head up or looking down causes dizziness;
- loss of scalp, hair, baldness, shaved head, skin grafts;
- possible hearing impairment and damage to ear;
- physical exhaustion—require one to two rests a day.

Cognitive Problems:

- short-term memory problems;
- attention problems; loses track of conversation, both as listener and as speaker;
- new learning problems—overloads easily, shuts off to cope, can't remember new details;
- attention problem—easily distracted, noise/activity/visual upsets;
- mental exhaustion after short application of one to one-and-a-half hours.

Emotional Problems:

- flatness—range of emotions now happy, sad, flatness, anger, frustration, depression; not enough joy/laughter;
- phobias—fear of further surgery, hospitalization, hitting head, falling, anything overhead falling on me;
- cry easily and inappropriately—over other people's problems, over sad things, fears, worries, phobias;
- loss of self-confidence;
- loss of independence; isolation; not driving;
- regular nightmares/bad dreams/bad daydreams— near-deaths, fears, horrible accident scenarios everywhere, and by/with everything;
- losses—not the way I was; not as "good or with it" as I was;

- shame of damage to head, hair, scalp; humiliation;
- depression, despondence—things going badly too long;
- loss of self-image, appearance issues; feel invisible;
- loss of femininity;
- loss of sex drive;
- dealing with feelings of going from forty-three-year-old woman to eighty-five-year-old one;
- changed personality—who am I now? What is my personality?

Other Losses and Problems:

- can't lay on right side—rod in hip painful after a few minutes; pillow presses on area of missing skull bone, dizziness;
- lost days due to extensive length of hospital stays—three months, plus three weeks, plus three weeks;
- head bandage, inconvenience, appearance, psyche—always had bangs and full head of beautiful shiny hair—gone;
- always aware of head problems—on alert to avoid possible injurious situations (hitting head, bumping head, being bumped or elbowed); hyper-vigilance;
- hobbies—gardening, dog walking, travelling restricted/hampered;
- now must always wear glasses (before, only for driving, and I hate glasses);
- the need to plan my life/leisure around physical,

emotional, cognitive limitations, problems, and weaknesses; loss of spontaneity;

- length of recuperation—two years and counting.

That's what I came up with at the time. I am working hard on learning to cope with these and new issues as they develop.

The accident changed my life completely. The injuries, while now for the most part healed in medical terms, are impacting on my life two-and-a-half years later, and many will always be a challenge. Brain injury lasts a lifetime.

The brain injury, while the most visually undetectable, remains the most pervasive of all. That is the nature of most brain injuries.

It's now three-and-a-half years following the accident, and Doug and I are watching a film in which the opening scene shows a young girl riding her horse up an icy hill. The horse loses its footing, begins panicking, and slips, rearing up, legs flailing, and making that horrible, gut-wrenching cry of panic as it struggles. The next scene shows a close-up of the horse's leg coming down hard on the frozen ground, splitting, breaking bone, and spewing blood. That's it. I, too, begin slipping; slipping into the terror that was my accident. I begin sobbing, stifling it so moviegoers cannot hear me. Eyes closed, I listen to the honk and roar of an approaching truck onscreen, and the horror cry of the rearing horse, which has slid onto the highway below and is now being crushed by the truck.

I am reduced to sheer sobbing fear, safe in my theatre seat beside Doug.

∽

You can take a tremendous load off your mind by taking inventory and getting your thoughts down on paper, such as I did, by making a list of my problems, complaints, and difficulties. It helps crystallize the big whys: why you are feeling ill; why you are feeling frustrated; why you are sad or depressed. Trust me, the act of writing it all down is very difficult; I was often in tears, but it is worth it. Do it.

By knowing why you are acting and feeling as you do (and what it is, exactly, you are feeling) you are able to step back and say to yourself, "No wonder I'm miserable and having such a hard time. Look at what I'm dealing with on a daily basis. All in all, I'm coping fairly well!" Give yourself a big pat on the back—you deserve one.

There is another reason to make a list; it has to do with legal implications of your illness or accident. Your lawyer may need this information for your case, or you may find it useful to have if you're required to undergo a neuro-psychological or physical assessment for insurance purposes. The information contained on this well thought-out list may prove invaluable.

It also helps if you can share your list with your caregiver, spouse, older children, or a trusted friend. By helping them understand your situation and weak areas, they are able to assist you in ways that can make a significant difference in your day-to-day existence. It also helps enlist a little sympathy. And, sometimes, there's nothing wrong with that.

❧ The Pain—Blockout

It happens so quickly. One split second and it's over. If it's minor, you may remember most of it. If it's major, you'll thankfully remember none of it. The accident. And the pain.

I had looked both ways before stepping off the curb. Halfway across the street I glanced up at the traffic signal ahead displaying the little man that meant "walk." It was then it happened. That horrible moment—the accident—that would change the rest of my life.

Did I feel a thing? No. I didn't feel the full-size van crush into my body, lift and throw me with its momentum 20 feet ahead. I didn't feel the hard landing, nor the tires ride over my body. No pain.

I awoke to perceive a crowd, utter some words, then sense a wet stickiness inside my coat sleeve. Words shouted from somewhere in the crowd, "Look at the tire tracks down her!" began a logical thought process in me which deduced, "something's horribly wrong here." With that realization, a surge of dread flooded through my body, followed by a sudden, sinking weakness. All auxiliary power was beginning to shut down.

No pain. Not yet.

My emergency power now took over, that fight or flight struggle for life that lies buried deep within us all. A no-frills reptilian brain. It took over and shut down all non-essential services, one by one.

Memories of visual, auditory, and tactile sensations of the moment were all relegated to some mysterious, dark internal safe. Overload experiences were shunted expediently out of the way, while all essential services—the nuts and bolts of survival—took all the focus and energy my traumatized body possessed.

Extreme pain is an overload sensation that, too intense to keep in that dark internal safe, reverberates throughout the body, penetrating every living cell. There it stays for months, perhaps years. Thankfully, your mind doesn't remember this pain, but your body does. It experienced it, and for the rest of your life this pain is part of you, changing you in ways both obvious and subtle.

Many patients I've talked with over the past few years relate the same tale. Survivors. They survived awful accidents, terrible injuries and disfigurements and they all "can't remember" the initial pain. The most horrible parts are blocked out; weak, fragmented memories are all they have. The worst minutes, hours, and days of their lives are like missing pieces of a puzzle. Mysteries trapped inside a ravaged body.

Memories of pain too lethal to remember.

Indeed, a merciful blessing.

∾ Therapists

When you acquire brain or orthopedic injuries, you also acquire therapists. I acquired a variety. There were hospital therapists, home care therapists, private therapists, occupational therapists, physical therapists, cognitive therapists, and clinical psychologist (therapist). There was also a logical progression of these.

While in the hospital Rehab Ward, I underwent the basics of physical therapy. The therapist's goal was to get me to the point that I could suffer a short walk with the aid of a cane and climb a short flight of steps. This took me two months. The highlight of this therapy was when a nurse, not having seen me for several days, observed me struggling down the hall with my cane. As I passed by, she commented on my progress. Since it's always good strategy to look on the lighter side of your hospital situation, I said, "Watch this! I also do reverse." With that, I turned the cane handles around to face the other way and stepped tentatively backwards. This elicited a surprised laugh from her, and soon other nurses gathered to participate in the merriment.

Occupational therapy mostly involved assessing the extent of my brain damage, and jump-starting those areas that had been weakened. I did get square pegs, but thankfully, never tried putting them into round holes. There were lots of manual dexterity exercises to attempt (which proved difficult while healing a broken elbow and a broken brain), and some basic movements, such as shifting the body from side to side while standing to simulate kitchen activities like drying dishes and putting them into the cupboard.

Rehab wasn't optional in the Rehab Ward; you couldn't get out of attending these exercise sessions because, at the appointed time, the therapist came to your room and got you. I enjoyed the routines and the cognitive stuff was fun, so I was always ready and waiting. The therapists were happy and lively, while being extremely considerate and knowledgeable of their patients' physical, emotional, and cognitive situations. We were pushed, but not beyond our capabilities.

After release from hospital, Home Care therapists began visiting on a regular basis. Their purpose was to initiate rehabilitation by introducing simple exercises, both physical and cognitive, that I could do in my very weakened state, mostly from a lying or sitting position: simple stretching and resistance exercises for the arms and legs, some walking and stand-up-sit-down training, exercises for the face muscles, and some visual scanning and memory exercises. One day the physical therapist scribbled some words on a piece of paper, held it up in front of my face, and asked what I saw. She'd written, "Opportunity is nowhere." I read aloud, "Opportunity is nowhere."

"Look again," she said. Slowly, the real message she offered appeared to me as I read, "Opportunity is now here."

Karen, the visiting occupational therapist, an energetic woman with a very expressive face and voice, got me up and out of the house on my walker to the garden, helping me resume some basic gardening activities. I needed to see the flowers, smell the freshly turned earth, and feel the sun.

A large portion of the therapists' time was spent giving me moral support, for in those early days of rehabilitation there was much pain, frustration, and tears. Now, "WHOA" were the words written on the sheet of paper for me and held up in front of my face. "Slow down, stop, rest!" was the therapist's message, as she tried to convince me that after such a traumatic accident healing goes slowly, and resting is a part of the healing process and of learning to adapt to my new limitations.

After Home Care visits ran out, I was taken by a Community Care driver four times a week to a private physiotherapy clinic. The clinic's job was to increase my strength, stamina, balance, and treat any resulting pain. Although less personal attention was received in this busy clinic, it was an opportunity to exercise and socialize in a safe and more normal environment. The therapist expected me to work hard, but was also aware that slow, steady progress was the best. Even the trip there and back was a cognitive exercise in social interaction and I enjoyed great conversations with Gerry, the driver, and his wife Helen.

Next came the exercise therapists, who designed an individualized exercise program to build on my previous achievements, in the comfort and privacy of my own home. The thing that bothered me the most was my low tolerance for any change to the exercise program. Eventually, it was explained to me that, when you have a brain injury, any physical, mental, or emotional stimulus is magnified. Noise seems louder. Lights seem brighter. Activity seems busier. An increase of 1 pound in hand-weights seems like an increase of 10 pounds, and so on. Because of this, I worked very hard and made steady but very slow progress. Regardless, Kim and Brenda (or "physio-terrorists," as I jokingly referred to them) became friends, and they too, had their share of consoling me during my emotional spells.

Now, three years post-accident, I have joined a health club. The personal trainer meets me there, and she will gradually (very gradually, as my strength and stamina increase) introduce me to the club equipment, and oversee my progress while monitoring pain and problems.

During all this, not only did my physical body need rehabilitation, so did my state of mind. The accident drastically changed all aspects of my life, so I regularly visited a clinical psychologist. Carol's job was to guide me through all the stages of loss, help me develop coping strategies for the problems I'm left with, and instill in me the confidence to accept my condition and move on. Starting out with weekly visits, over a three-year period I have progressed to monthly visits. Even on those days when I'm feeling fairly positive when arriving for my session, I end up crying over another of the myriad issues that bother me. Nevertheless, it's a very safe place to cry. There's a lot of fear, hurt, disappointment, frustration, and pain buried inside a lot of us; crying helps get it out. Honest, it's OK to cry.

Other therapists I have known and loved are: the brain injury day-planner therapist, who helped me customize a day-planner system for my special needs, and dried my tears from time to time; and the Therapeutic Touch practitioner (a veritable angel named Donna), who used her craft to help relax and heal me, as well as comfort me when more tears worked their way out.

As different as each individual therapist is, they have one common denominator: nothing makes them happier than to see a patient who applies himself to his exercises to the best of his abilities—patients who listen to their therapists and take heed of their advice. Therapists are very goal oriented, and they like to see progress, no matter how small, in their patients; they truly want to help you get well. Too often they are disheartened by patients who refuse to put a solid effort into their therapy, who prefer to give up on themselves by not participating in their own healing.

Are you that type of patient? I hope not. Although you may think momentarily that you are victorious over the system, you have unwittingly surrendered to your particular affliction. You are the loser, always, in this give-up game. Don't play it.

∞ Hair

Shiny hair—our crowning glory—is a barometer of good health. In the hospital, my hair, or rather the lack of it, was a major concern of mine.

In the operating room following my accident, the neurosurgeon removed a 3" x 2" oval of skull bone to allow expansion room for my swelling brain. An arc along the right side of my head, from above the ear and down behind it to the nape of the neck, had been shaved for surgery.

As a general rule, when surgeons, doctors, and nurses are struggling to save your life, they do not pay much attention to your hairstyle. Mercifully, they left me a fringe of bangs and a flap of long hair on top to hang down and over the shaved area. Post-surgery, this flap of hair was tied in a perky topknot perched upon my head.

It wasn't until I moved from Intensive Care to Critical Care that I became consciously aware of my hair. The topknot gave me somewhat of a punk look; others told me I looked like Pebbles. I thought it gave me attitude. Having never before worn my hair up like that, it was a novelty, as well as a source of irritation; irritation because it tugged at my scalp, and because it just looked irritating to me. I was used to a blunt-cut, reminiscent of the '60s and '70s "That Girl" style.

The first hair "washing" was administered ten days post-accident (New Year's Eve) by my sister-in-law Vici, who arrived at bedside equipped with a wide-tooth comb and baby wipes. Removing the elastic band from around the topknot and untangling my hair was not a simple proposition; it had become hopelessly tangled. After a quick trip to the store to fetch some detangler and conditioner, she began the comb-out, which proved time-consuming and painful. Baby-wipes were used to dry bath my hair, removing some dirt and bits of dried blood that had accumulated from the accident and surgery. A final combing returned my hair to some semblance of normal.

Real relief didn't come until two days later when, in answer to my pleas, a nurse performed a 3:00 a.m. bed-shampoo. What pleasure it was to feel the warm water and gentle massaging fingers on my scalp, and to hear the splashing sound the water made. Heavenly! It took six rinses until the water ran clear; my hair was that dirty. This was all performed while I lay on my back, with no spilled water wetting the bed, which I thought to be quite a miracle. This simple act made such a difference to my sense of well being. Having my hair washed was a mood lifter; I felt more human and cared for.

Three weeks later, after I was moved to the city hospital and was slightly more mobile, I began to notice my hair was falling out. Not a strand here and there, but a constant shedding of hair, after hair, after hair.

I'd comb my hair and have a comb full. I'd brush my hair and have a brush full. I'd sit up in bed and look at my pillow, and I'd have a pillow full. There was hair on the pillowcase, on the bedsheets, in my towel, and on my nightgown. It was horrendous.

I became obsessed, telling the nurses and doctors my hair was falling out.

"It's the anaesthetic; it's the trauma; it's the lying in bed all the time," they'd say.

Well, it was all that, plus the anti-seizure drug I was receiving, which not only caused hair loss on my head, but at the same time increased hair growth on my arms and legs. This was all too distressing. And nowhere was the hair so apparent as it was at bath time.

Bath time at the hospital, during that point in my recovery, consisted of being chair-lifted into a huge tub filled with tepid water in a chilly room. Once bathing began, the hair on my arms was now so dark and long that I entertained myself swishing my arms back and forth in the water, while watching the changing hair patterns on my arms—quite mesmerizing. When the tub was drained, the hair lost during shampooing coated the bottom of the tub; my eyes transfixed upon this sight with horror, as the automated chair lifted me up, up, up, out of the tub, swung me clear, then lowered me onto the cold bathroom tiles. After a quick dry down performed by the nurse, I was bundled into the wheelchair and taken back to the room.

My obsession continued, but in the months after I left the hospital a wonderful thing happened. Slowly—as I ate better, got healthier, was weaned off some drugs, and sat up more in bed—my hair loss lessened. The shaved areas on my head began to grow in, and I took the razor to my arms and legs.

A year following the accident, my hair looked quite normal, although the shaved area on my head was still shorter than the rest. Now all I had to worry about hair-wise, was the next surgery to have my bone piece, or "bone flap" as they called it, replaced in the side of my skull. I wondered how much of my head they would shave this time. Save the bangs, and leave me a nice long flap of hair again, please. I wasn't asking for much.

Four months later, in May '96, it was time to have the bone put back into the side of my head—a cranioplasty, they called it. The surgery comes and goes. Happily, not a lot of hair is removed, and I'm left with bangs and most of my hair. The side had been shaved again, so the scalp could be pulled back to expose the brain during surgery, the bone piece replaced, and the skin sewn back down. The post-surgical look is one of a large white bandage taped to the side of my head. With clever combing, I minimize the big bandage effect by hiding most of it under my hair. (I didn't really "hide" anything, but trying to, did make me feel better.)

Things did not continue smoothly. Some time later, due to an unfortunate incident during a dressing change at the hospital, I developed a large hematoma on the surgical site. Released from hospital to recuperate at home in the country, I agonized as the large, bloated bruise progressed to an infection, attacking the replaced bone piece, and killing the skin covering it. I'm pestered by flies landing on my head dressing, drawn to the oozing pus and rotting flesh underneath. It was as disgusting and as upsetting as it sounds.

After two months it became evident that, despite massive antibiotic therapy, further surgery is required to remove the infected bone flap to prevent possible brain infection. Doug and I jokingly coin this scheduled operation an anti-cranioplasty; basically, reversing the cranioplasty they did before. What I learned next was a nightmare.

The neurosurgeon informed me that he now had to enlist the assistance of a plastic surgeon for the upcoming operation. Not only is all the skin on the side of my head dead, but the bone flap is infected too, requiring: (1) removal of the infected bone patch; (2) removal of the dead skin from the side of my head (all layers); (3) rotation of the healthy scalp (all skin layers) from the top of my head to the right side; and (4) grafting a layer of skin from my thigh to the top of my scalped head.

As frightening as it sounded, I knew the surgery had to be done. I resigned myself to the fact my head would be totally shaved for surgery this time, and that I would look positively bizarre for a long time. My life with shiny, long, chestnut hair and bangs would end. It was the only life I'd known.

The second surgery is done July '96. Initially I'm left with a huge head dressing, very top-heavy and uncomfortable, inspiring Doug to tease in a whining, pleading voice "I am not Marge Simpson, I am a human being...." That comment sent me into a laughing fit. We hurriedly made a sign with this new motto, taping it to the wall across from my bed.

Eventually, it was time for the unveiling.

The entire medical team assembled to witness the mountain of gauze and dressing pads being removed. Although I could not see it, my exposed head was ugly, bloody, scabby, and discoloured, and I had been completely shaved, scalped, grafted, stapled, and stitched. The doctors, surgeons, and nurses stared at me, blank-faced, speechless. In response, I bowed my head, embarrassed by my grotesqueness.

In the days and weeks that passed, my head was cleaned, the staples and stitches removed, and I was left with a moonscape—a large scalped, sunken area at the top and back of my head, with mountainous hunks of red scabs and a few craters.

Doug warned me not to look at it—it would be too depressing for me—and I didn't look for a long time. It was easy not to, as I still had dressings covering my head. Eventually, the larger dressings were removed. The Home Care nurse replaced them with a 4"x 4" gauze pad on top, to protect the scalped scalp under the cotton turban I'd started wearing. In the following days I coined the phrase "doily" to refer to that tiny piece of delicate white gauze.

Sneaking a peek (sans glasses) here and there of my moonscape reflected in the mirror during dressing changes, slowly conditioned me for the imminent unveiling. That occurred shortly after the home care nurse and surgeons removed the last of the mountainous scabs during various visits at home and to the hospital.

I stared into the mirror. A bit of fuzz had begun to grow on two-thirds of my head, but the scalped and grafted area was sickly and huge.

In the following weeks my hair began to grow, but I kept my bald patch covered. Selected people who saw me said I looked cute—like a pixie—and that I looked good in short hair. I gazed at them with astonishment and gratitude, and later started to think maybe I didn't look *that* bad. The fashion magazines were picturing models with short, buzzed cuts; maybe I'd be all right with this. Just maybe. And look, the hair on the upper left side was about

1 '" and was starting, naturally, to lean over onto the bald area to eventually cover it.

In the meantime, I'd collected an assortment of turbans, scarves, kerchiefs, and hats, and was beginning to think about hairpieces. People said I looked cosmopolitan, exotic, like an old-time film star in my turbans. Their comments both surprised and entertained me, but I knew that underneath my headgear there was only a 4"x 4" gauze doily and a lot of chutzpah keeping me sane.

The plastic surgeon said that over time—a long time—the scalped/bald/grafted area will reduce to about half the size it is now, and the hair will be long enough around it to comb and style for maximum camouflage. He added, there are operations to surgically minimize and even remove the grafted site, but they are not simple, not without danger for me.

Three-and-a-half months after surgery I sat trying to heal my still seeping and leaking head, and tried to visualize myself with a full head of shiny chestnut hair—something I knew would never happen. I would always have that large bald spot.

One day when someone said to me, "You need a tidy-up haircut," I laughed. Reluctantly, I put a reminder in my day-planner to call the stylist and set the appointment. Somehow, getting it cut again just didn't sit well with me.

I wouldn't be able to say, "A little off the top" (I have nothing on the top), so instead I'd say, "A little off the sides, please."

∾

It's almost four years post-accident, and after several halfhearted attempts to "look at wigs" I finally decide to give it a serious try. Although still paper thin, the skin graft on the top of my head has toughened-up enough to consider hairpieces. Increasing my head-wear options is what interests me. I'm bored of the hat look—whether it's a baseball cap, canvas hat, straw hat, turban, toque, or beret.

Trying on a wig was a humiliating experience. First I had to s-t-r-e-t-c-h an extremely tight nylon stocking cap onto my head and tuck all my hair up underneath it. Then I had to sit looking at my hideous (to me) image in the overly-lit mirror. Next I endured the onslaught of "let's see what this one looks like" assortment of wig types and styles. All of them had one thing in common— they made me look like either Herb Tarlick from WKRP in Cincinnati, or a person with a really bushy cat perched atop their skull. "Get that off my head!" I'd whine at the salon owner.

Eventually I decided on a curly chestnut fall attached to a black hairband. It wasn't a Dolly Parton wig, but it came pretty close. Instantly I had Big Hair. Doug insisted I wear the fall home, knowing if I didn't start wearing it right away, once we got home it would be tossed into a closet and left there.

I don't know why Doug and I named the fall "Betty," but we did. Betty became my alter ego who sometimes compelled me to wear very short skirts. Doug would ask, "Are you taking Betty to town today?" meaning, "Are you wearing your fall?"

"Yes, Betty's going to town today," I'd reply.

Betty got more attention than I usually did. More

men would smile at me. Teenage boys would notice me. Some of our older male friends would smile a little brighter, or hold me a little longer while greeting me or bidding farewell.

My brother remarked, "What the heck you got on your head?" then later teased, "Hey, Annette. Oh, Miss Funicello!"

"Nice do, Bev," commented our young male neighbour.

Some female friends were surprised and happy for me. "It takes twenty years off you!" they'd say in a backward compliment. Others stared at me with a stunned look on their faces, never having seen me in curly hair before. One girlfriend wanted a Betty, too. Another friend tried on Betty but was transformed into Ski Bunny Heather instead.

As Betty "got out" more, I began noticing a strange phenomenon. While paying for a drink one day at the coffee shop, I happened to glance over my shoulder at a curvy blonde lady with Big Hair. Our eyes met and held. Time stood still. She smiled at me; I smiled at her, nodded, and waved. After that, many times during my travels I'd look up and notice a voluptuous-haired lady staring knowingly in my direction. And always I'd smile and nod back. Was it that she knew I was wearing a fall; did she think I knew she was wearing a fall; or did she conclude I knew the secrets that all Big Hair ladies learn about life and love?

I had unofficially become a member of the Big Hair Sorority.

Surely the sweetest comment I received was when Doug first saw me with Betty on and said, "You know, you remind me of how you looked in that photograph of us at our friend's wedding twenty-six years ago."

I think Betty is worth her weight in gold.

❧ Philosophy and Religion

What happened to me, happened for a reason. In retrospect, after a lot of thinking and reading, I can say that.

However, in the first several months after the accident, all I could think about was "Why me? Why didn't this happen to a bad person—a murderer or a rapist? I'm a good person—why did it happen to me?"

When I returned home from the hospital three months after the accident, I phoned those friends and acquaintances who had showered me with cards and flowers, to thank them for their thoughtfulness and to let them know I was home.

Many made comments such as:

"It wasn't your time to die."

"Your job on earth isn't finished yet."

"There's still more you have to do."

"You're so strong. You've got such inner strength."

I was puzzled at first, but later, after some thought, my delayed reactions to these statements were:

"What's this job on earth that's not finished yet?"

"What am I still supposed to do?"

"Strength? All I was doing, was trying to survive."

During one of my earliest public outings, I headed to the town library. There it was, a book titled, Why Me? Why This? Why Now? by Robin Norwood. It leapt off the shelf at me. Was this a coincidence? Or was this an act of synchronicity? I believe it was the latter.

After an absorbed two readings, a sort of calm settled on me. Suddenly everything I had experienced, or wondered about, or thought about with respect to spirituality since I was a young child, seemed to come into focus.

Everything made sense. Everything. Even my accident made sense.

I learned that everything happened the way it was supposed to that day. It happened to me for a reason. Not because I was "bad" or being punished, but because there was something I had to do or learn to advance on my spiritual journey or life path. I read that good things come out of bad things; a sort of healing happens. People grow, mature, and take a different path through life—for the good of themselves, for the good of the immediate family, for the good of the larger community.

I learned, too, that everything and everyone are connected, the activities of one person impacting on others, known or unknown, around them through infinity, all part of a greater interactive and interconnected plan.

Although we may weigh the pros and cons of an impending decision, the decision we make and the action we take is the only one we can—and it is, therefore, the right one for us. We end up doing "what we're supposed to do" in our journey through life.

During my convalescence, there was a lot of time to read and think. I read works by:

Robin Norwood: *Why Me? Why This? Why Now?;*
Betty J. Eadie: *Embraced by the Light;*
Deepak Chopra: *The Seven Spiritual Laws of Success;*
Julia Cameron: *The Artist's Way.*

I also listened to the cassette tape by Louise Hays, titled "Self-Healing."

Thinking about these philosophies, which are based on scientific and universal laws, helped speed up my healing process, crystallized my spiritual identity, and offered me understanding, confidence, and peace.

I would highly recommend Robin Norwood's book to anyone wrestling with "why me, why this, why now" feelings following an accident or during illness, or faced with any other puzzling life-crisis questions.

While not a religious person, I have always been a spiritual one. These teachings helped me tremendously during my illness.

In many of the darkest hours of my recovery I asked God for help, drinking in the power and the healing of his universal love around me—a force available to us all.

❧ The Dream: Accident Revisited

They say you remember everything; that all your experiences are locked inside, not only in your brain cells, but also in body cells. They even have a name for it—cellular memory—where the most horrible, traumatic, painful memories are stored. Too dangerous to be recalled at will, they are stored deep within your body's tissues, and muscles, and bones—hidden away. In time these memories may work themselves out, fragments escaping bit by bit, easing out in small manageable doses.

Sometimes these memory fragments connect to conscious memories and values, resurfacing at night into the brain's downloading, which we call dreaming.

It wasn't until twenty-seven months following the accident, that the first real memory of it and the emergency surgery emerged. There they were in my dream, bits of sensations, feelings, visions, fears, and experiences all interwoven into a grand play unfolding before me.

Months earlier my dreams were shorter and had common themes revolving around some traumatic aspect of the experience, but they did not deal with the actual accident. My red coat, cars/trucks, urgency, catastrophe, fears/lack of fear, and helplessness were all elements in those dreams.

But that morning of March '97, I awoke in a strange kind of grogginess. As I lay there images began to replay in my mind, and bit by bit, the dream pieced itself together for me one more time. Slowly I became aware of the importance of it all, in an eerie sort of uneasiness, sadness, and revelation.

I sat up, grabbed a pen, and wrote furiously in my bedside journal. Faster, before the details dissolve. The images were astounding, all neatly packaged into one strange, disturbing dream. As I wrote, tears dripped onto the pages. Powerful stuff, I thought. The first comprehensive recollection of my December 21/94 accident experience.

I am in the air, standing up on the front of a plane, I think, trying desperately to keep my balance as I am pushed forward through the air, all the while changing speed and height, arms flailing, balancing myself...

(Sensation of being pushed through the air after being hit by a van.)

...Now, I am seated beside Doug at the back of a large room or auditorium filled with people. Someone at the front is calling out names and handing out certificates or awards to people stepping forward. It is Dr. S., my neurosurgeon. The awards are to his staff it seems. But he is mumbling, and we can't be sure what he is saying.

(It's the operating room and staff are handing him instruments for surgery on me.)

Then the surgeon holds up a certificate which I think is for me, but we can't hear well, so we don't go up and get it. We all clap. After, as we leave, he is sitting off to the side of the room on a bench, totally exhausted. I say hi and something to the effect that not only was I a patient, but also a worker. He says there was one other person, and points to a list. There are initials beside only two people on the list, me and one other.

Doug and I leave the crowded room, but it's crowded outside, too. We get separated. I walk back and forth waiting outside, then realize I have no turban on. I reach up and feel the sparse hair combed over the top of my head to cover my bald spot. It seems so real, I can feel it—the hair and the bald scalp. I am wearing my red woolen winter coat, high heels and nylons. I pace back and forth for a while, then head back through the crowd.

(Bald spot is a more recent reference of scalp surgery one-and-a-half years post-accident. The clothes described are the ones I wore when hit by the van.)

There are very bright, stadium-like lights now, and I am walking through a milling crowd gathering, it seems, for some event, towards these bright overhead lights.

(References to the operating room filled with operating room staff, or recovery room.)

144

I still can't see Doug. I am aware of people around me and of the bright lights over me. A very tall man and someone else are behind me, and they comment on the "shiner"—perhaps the light bouncing off my oily, bald head.

(Doctors and my surgeon looking down at me as I lie on the operating table. The shiner refers to my very badly bruised and swollen head and body, but could also refer to my later scalp surgery and resulting bald spot.)

I keep looking for Doug, then leave the crowded area, walking away from the bright lights.

(Perhaps being wheeled through the hospital tunnel to another room.)

I walk and walk. I look down. I am carrying my purse or something in my left hand.

(When hit I was carrying a briefcase; or perhaps the reference is to medical equipment attached to my arm, hand, etc.)

I continue until I come to a park-like area and realize I am lost. Where is Doug? I keep walking. How will he find me here? A dappled brown, grouse-like bird rises up and flaps by overhead from the left, landing in a tree beside me to the right. I watch, then turn my head back and notice a rough-looking man with long, wavy, bedraggled hair and dark features. There is blood dripping down his face, arm, and hand. He walks by, looking at me in a menacing, foreboding way. He raises a bloody finger and points at the tree to the right. I look to the right and see a small, beautiful, delicate, almost iridescent green bird sitting in the tree now. Ethereal, otherworldly.

(Is this Jesus pointing out the transition of death to afterlife, a beautiful ethereal state?)

The man passes by, and I keep walking. Now I become aware of my danger and am beginning to tire. I look behind me at the bright lights far back in the distance, but turn and keep walking ahead.

(I turn away from "the light.")

I soon come to a street and decide to turn. As I leave the park, there are still some people walking and talking close behind me. The street is very dark and I am afraid. Cars pass.

(Being wheeled by hospital staff and nurses through hospital corridors. Other operating beds and people pass me.)

I soon come to a point where I have to decide which way to go. Ahead is a dark street lined with houses. To the left there appears to be a tunnel under what seems to be an apartment or building complex. There are bright lights at the end of this tunnel. I decide to go that way, towards the streetlights, I think, where I might find a cab and look for Doug.

(Decision—do I choose death, or do I choose life? I begin the path "towards the light," i.e., death.)

Now I am getting very tired walking in my heavy red coat and high heels, carrying my bag. I have walked so terribly far— but I must continue.

(I have been through so much, come so far, and am getting so very weary.)

The footsteps behind me are closer now. I begin to panic and think, "What if I fall down or they push me down, and I hit my head and die in this tunnel. How will Doug ever find me?"

(I am afraid of death, of Doug losing me, and of losing Doug.)

I stop, paralyzed, look again at the bright lights ahead, then wake up.

(I decide to live.)

❧

It is 6:00 a.m. on Saturday, March 8, 1997 and my dream is ripe with symbolism and memories; a luscious glimpse into my accident experience of December 21/94: a reference to my bald spot, a result of later surgeries; the sensations of feeling my hair and bare scalp so real, I must have actually reached up while dreaming and felt my head; references to a Christ figure showing me the transition from a mundane life (brown bird) to an exquisite afterlife (as an ethereal emerald bird); the white lights of death, which I flee from, then turn towards in exhaustion, but turn away from again to choose life at the last moment; the bright lights of operating rooms and hospital corridors, and surgeons bent over me; and always the searching for Doug.

❧

My psychologist listens to the dream intently, then comments about how close to death I must have been. I nearly died.

But I didn't.

Final Notes

ೕ In Retrospect

If you are seriously ill, there is simply no other place to be than in the hospital. Regardless of the seeming mistakes and assorted problems I encountered, plus the added complications of being on blood thinners, the truth is hospitals saved my life four times. The majority of things went right for me during my stays. With my many scars, injured psyche, and assorted foreign body parts (about thirty-three at last count), hospitals have literally kept me alive. For this, I owe them eternal thanks.

If you are facing hospitalization, keep in mind that you are ultimately responsible for your own healing, and you do have to look out for yourself. Ask questions; get them answered, even if it's as simple as asking what pills they're giving you each time. (I got the wrong pills a couple times, but then again the chances for error was high—I was given pills at least three times a day, over a period of several months.) Demand attention when you truly need it. Trust your gut feeling or intuition. Don't be afraid to stand up for your rights. Doctors and nurses are not infallible—they're human. They can and do make mistakes, but don't fear: most things will be done correctly. Take care of yourself. Don't be shy. If you are, have someone with you who's not intimidated by medical professionals and who will get you the information and care you need.

Many times during my long recovery I cried about my situation, feeling defeated, frustrated, and wondering what kind of life lay ahead. But many times I laughed.

I laughed, not at the situation as a whole, because in fact it was quite serious, but at many of the various aspects of it. Those funny bits and pieces and moments that are part of everyday life were there, too, at the hospital.

Hospital life is like Life. It possesses the same ups and downs, the same highs and lows. To present one side only in this book, either the good or the bad, would have been untruthful on my part and I would have done you a disservice. My point is, despite some very serious medical predicaments—heart surgery, a near-fatal accident, and complications—I survived. I went through the bad stuff, experienced a lot of the good stuff, and came out the other end alive. At times it seemed the situation was endless. Time dragged. But as the saying goes, this too shall pass. One by one the days went by; things got better.

At home, as I struggled to return my life to some semblance of normal, I saw that the best way to cope was to look for the funny aspects of my new situation. Many times it was impossible to see the bright side, so I reached out to friends, relatives, therapists, doctors, or anyone who could help me. I believe everyone can find someone to help them through their toughest moments. The key is to know you need help and to ask for it. Seek and you shall find.

And amazingly, every once in a while help mysteriously found me at the precise moment I needed it the most, without my even having to ask for it. Divine intervention? Definitely. Knock and the door shall be opened.

I decided early on after the accident, that it was important to focus my energy into getting well. Blaming the driver who caused my problems would not make me better; it would only confuse my thinking and compromise my healing. It was the right decision. At a time of such mental and physical upheaval, clear thinking, a goal, and dogged determination was the right combination for survival.

As I near the five-year anniversary of my accident, I think about how my life has changed. The major change is that now I cry only rarely.

At home in the country, life goes on. It's not the same life I had before the accident, but it's my new life and it has many positive sides. The big plus is that I have more time to devote to the things I love.

Take gardening, for instance. I've set up small, manageable gardens throughout the property. I work slowly and only on the most pleasant of days, moving from one garden to the next as my energy level dictates.

I walk each day accompanied by one, and sometimes even two, of my dogs. We take our time and dally along the way, whether it's to look at the clouds, a wildflower, a chipmunk on a cedar rail fence, a cornfield rustling in the breeze, or a breathtaking sunset.

I write short stories or work on my next book. I occasionally volunteer at the local brain injury association. I spend more time with my sister, sometimes helping her with her reading, playing cards or board games with her, or taking her on short outings. I have lunch with friends from time to time, some old friends and some new.

I take the train to Toronto to visit Mom and Dad every once in a while. I worked on a family tree, a project I'd previously only thought about doing one day "when I had the time," and presented it at my parents' sixtieth anniversary dinner. Our family is closer now than it has ever been, and I believe it is a direct result of my health

problems and the resulting appreciation of the precious-
ness of life. A major shifting of priorities.

I've taken some night school courses to brush up on
my high school French and to learn computer basics.

I've taken several short holidays with Doug, with the
goal of working up to a full week's vacation one day soon.

I'm enjoying many aspects of my new life and, while
life isn't the same as it was before the accident and I miss
many of the things I used to do, it's a good life. And
although I'm not the same as I was before the accident, I'm
slowly evolving, becoming the person I'll be tomorrow,
just like you are, just like everyone is always evolving. I
look forward to the future with hope.

I've learned many lessons along the way, the type of
lessons learned only through the experience of extreme
hardship: lessons like living for today and not dwelling in
the past; believing in yourself and always trying to do
your best every day; being brave enough to try something
new; living in a less-than-perfect situation, but finding a
way to love it anyway; viewing the suffering of others
with genuine heart-felt compassion; being thankful for the
basic goodness of people, and for those selfless souls who
day after day, whether in a medical setting or at home,
care for the ill and the frail.

I hope you have found my adventures and the tales of
others related in this book of some interest, help, amusement, or comfort, and that you have learned something
about the hospital experience facing many long-term
patients. Appropriate medical intervention, dedicated caregivers, courage, and the curative powers of faith, hope, and
laughter are contributing factors for successful recovery.

Most of all, I hope you have learned that the human body is truly a wondrous creation, designed to survive, to heal, and to thrive.

I don't know what tomorrow will bring—who does? That's life's adventure.

Let the adventure begin.

Appendix
Strategies and Suggestions

❧ Hospital Strategies

If you have to be in the hospital, you might as well make the best of it. This statement is so blatantly obvious it eludes many patients. You are going there to get well and the doctors, nurses, and surgeons are all going to help you. They can do everything in the world they know how to do, but if you're not going to help yourself get well, too, then your healing won't be as successful as it could be.

What can you do? Several things:

1. You can do what you're told. Oddly enough, many patients don't follow orders. If you're told not to scratch your wound, don't scratch it. If you're told to lie still and don't try to get up, lie still and don't try to get up. If you're told to do some simple exercises in bed to help facilitate your healing, do them.

2. You can look out for yourself. The hospital is a busy place and hospital staff is overworked. Things get overlooked, details lost, mistakes made. If the doctor tells you to wait three days before having a shower, and the nurse prepares you for a shower on the second day, question it. If you see a pill in your pill cup that looks unfamiliar, ask what it is and who prescribed it. If you believe something's gone wrong in your healing schedule or a piece of equipment appears to be malfunctioning, bring it to someone's attention.

3. You can think healing thoughts. Help your body heal by telling yourself the medical staff are touching you with

healing hands, and their procedures are being accepted by your body, promoting healing and wellness. In your mind's eye, see your body mending itself. See yourself healthy and whole again—the way you want to be.

4. You can ask for emotional or spiritual help. Although you may be going through some of the most difficult times in your life, you have to maintain a positive outlook. If you are finding that difficult, ask the nurse to recommend someone to talk with you. A few moments with a nurse, therapist, or pastor can alleviate much of your distress and give you renewed hope. So can that talk with The Creator you've been putting off for so long. "Please help me, God," are words I heard more than once.

5. You can divert your attention. When we change our focus from a negative self-interest (worry, fear) to a positive outside interest (compassion, love), we can benefit our own healing. Look at the patient in the next bed. Are they lonely, hurting, or afraid? Kind words and thoughtful actions from you, not only give you a break from your suffering, they also help alleviate the suffering of another. It's healing that benefits the two of you. Another by-product is it reduces boredom and speeds the passage of time.

6. You can maintain some of your daily rituals. If you like putting on makeup every day, why not do it in the hospital? It will make you feel better. If you like to have a warm cup of milk or soothing herbal tea at night as a precursor to sleep, by all means arrange to have that provided. If you never miss a favourite TV program, arrange for a rental TV. If you love looking at plants or sitting in the sun, find a way to accommodate that, too. Anything that

makes you more comfortable or feel more at home helps your healing.

7. You can laugh. You've heard of laughter being the best medicine, and, well, it probably is. Find something to laugh about. Laughter massages your internal organs and releases feel-good chemicals in your brain that promote healing. As horrible as your situation may be, there's probably a little bit of irony, a little bit of slapstick, a little bit of, "You'll never believe what happened," either happening to you now, or going on around you. Seek out that humour. You may have to dig really, really deep at times to find it, but believe me, it's there. And it's worth it.

Here's an example of what I mean. After my second head surgery in which they cut away more of my skull bone, removed dead putrefied skin from the side of my head, cut and rotated my scalp, and slapped on a skin graft, I emerged from surgery with layer upon layer of white gauze piled up (way up) high on top of my head. It weighed a ton, felt lopsided, and looked preposterous. Finding the humour in the situation, Doug made me a sign that said, "I am not Marge Simpson" (A TV cartoon personality who sports a mountain of blue hair), "I am a human being," and taped it to the wall across from my hospital bed. Every time I looked at it I had to smile. I knew I was grotesque under the dressing, but that didn't stop me from laughing at the absurdity of the bandage itself. Situation hopeless—bandage really, really funny.

❧

The moral to this story is five-fold: never give up on yourself; realize you're responsible for your own healing;

look out for yourself; find the humour in your situation; and put your concentrated best efforts into getting well.

❧ Patient Checklist

The following suggestions are designed for the patient; if you're the caregiver, some items may apply to you as well.

- Start a hospital diary. Keep track of what happens and what the doctors say. Keep track of your feelings and emotions. Journalling is an excellent outlet.

- Bring a book, cards, a game, or a manageable craft project.

- Leave jewellery and money at home. A nominal amount of cash may be helpful for the tuck shop cart that comes along, or for a bite from the cafeteria.

- Rent a TV if bored. Rent earphones, too, if your roommate is not a TV fan; or keep the volume low.

- Bring a small transistor radio from home. Bring the earphones, too, so as not to disturb other patients.

- Ladies, take your blush and lipstick. Also, your favourite shampoo and conditioner. Use them. They will help you feel better.

- Bring your special pillow or other comfort item.

- Bring any special teas you like; relaxing varieties include chamomile or sleepytime blends.

- Bring your good luck charm, inspirational, or spiritual materials. Bring anything that gives you hope, courage, or comfort.

- Make a list of the pills you take, the dosage and how often, and take it with you. Leave your own pills at home, as the hospital will supply your medications.

- Take your medical information: a list of past surgeries and dates, major illnesses, health problems, drug allergies, food sensitivities, and any other pertinent information regarding your current illness or accident. You will be asked these details often. Better yet, take photocopies of it to hand out when asked.

- Take your health card and hospital card.

- Take a list of friends and family phone numbers and your phone charge card.

- Make sure you can reach your bed buzzer to summon a nurse if needed.

- Do what the nurses tell you to do.

- Do what the doctors tell you to do.

- Check that the right pills are in your pill cup. Question the nurse if something seems wrong.

- Find out what post-operative bed exercises you'll be doing. Practice them now. Learn some stretches or isometric exercises to do. Ask what activities you should refrain from.

- Keep track of what the doctors tell the nurses

regarding your care. You may have to remind the nurses to get these things done. Don't be afraid to remind them.

- If you're allowed to walk (alone or with help), start walking a lap or two around the hospital corridors as soon as you are able. Muscle atrophy and resulting weakness sets in quickly within several days' bed rest and inactivity. Activity helps prevent digestive sluggishness as well.

- Look for the humour in your situation or around you. It can be found, and it is good medicine.

- Give yourself a pat on the back, you deserve it.

❧ Visitor and Caregiver Checklist

These items are written with the visitor and caregiver in mind.

- Visit as often as you can.

- If the patient is especially debilitated, keep your visits short unless you are the caregiver; in that case, they need your moral support. Just being there—holding their hand or stroking their brow—is wonderfully beneficial.

- If you can't visit, a phone call may do. Remember to let the phone ring many times—hospital patients are notoriously slow moving.

- If you say you will visit on a certain day, try to keep your promise. If you can't make it, call and explain when you will be able to visit. Patients often feel forgotten and look forward to visits with much anticipation.

- If a caregiver, check in at the desk each day you visit to get an update on patient condition, treatment concerns, needs, etc.

- Bring an interesting or funny story and greeting from those unable to visit; perhaps recent vacation photos of family and friends.

- Bring a small gift or surprise; if homemade goodies, check any diet restrictions.

- If you know their interests, take a current copy of a favourite magazine.

- Any special diet concerns? Any diet supplementation required?

- Be creative. Perhaps you can solve the patient's hospital problem or concern with a bit of originality.

- With nurse's approval, take the patient on a wheelchair trip around the halls, or to the TV room, or to the cafeteria for a change of scenery. You may have to sign a register at the nurse's station with "out" and "return" times.

- What activities are to be restricted or avoided when released from hospital?

- What activities are OK? Which are beneficial?

- Any bathing concerns or restrictions?

- Special care of wounds? How often should dressing changes be done?

- Medications—what and when? They will give you prescriptions to have filled. Any precautions?

- Need special equipment? Where available? Who organizes them—you or Home Care? Who pays?

- Ask the doctors/dietician of any special diet requirements for when the patient returns home.

- Are there any follow-up appointments with surgeon or specialist required after patient's release from hospital?

- Tell the patient you'll pray for them and do it, even if it's simply, "Please help Mary get better," said with compassion and love. Prayer is a powerful force. It doesn't matter whether or not you're religious; everyone can be spiritual and tap into universal healing energies.

- Ask others to pray for the patient.

- If a caregiver, take some time out to care for yourself. Talk to someone you're comfortable with to help share the emotional load.

- Give yourself a pat on the back. You deserve it.

View from the Bedpan was nominated
for the 2003 Stephen Leacock
Memorial Medal for Humour

—